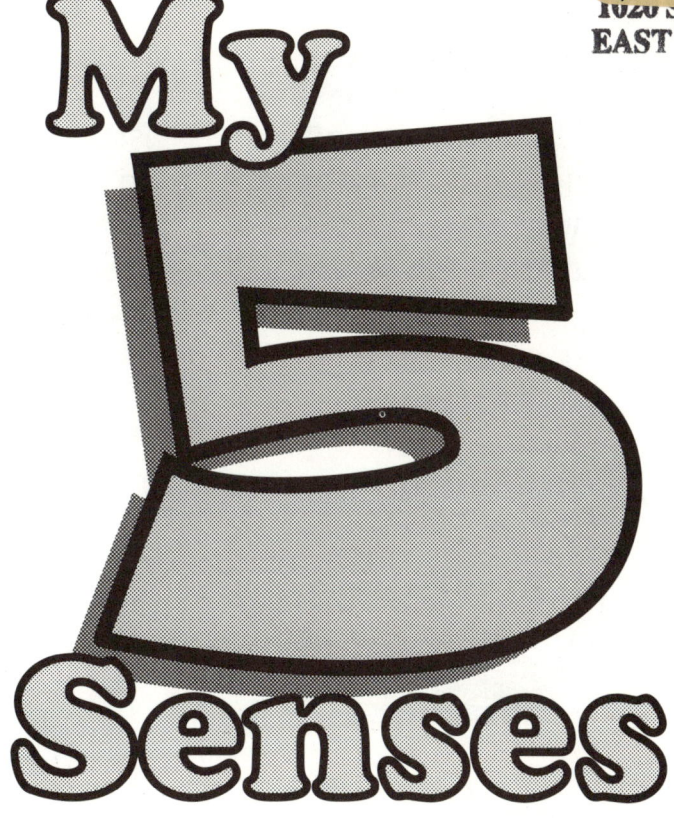

My 5 Senses

Gloria A. Truitt

Illustrated by Ed Koehler

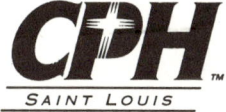

Scripture quotation: NEW INTERNATIONAL VERSION™ © 1973, 1978, 1984 by the International Bible Society. Used by permission of Zondervan.

Copyright © 1994 Concordia Publishing House
3558 S. Jefferson Avenue, St. Louis, MO 63118-3968
Manufactured in the United States of America

Teachers may reproduce pages for classroom use only. Parents may reproduce pages when necessary for the completion of an activity.

All rights reserved. Except as noted above, no part of this publication may be reproduced, stored in a retrieval system, or transmitted, in any form or by any means, electronic, mechanical, photocopying, recording, or otherwise, without the prior written permission of Concordia Publishing House.

1 2 3 4 5 6 7 8 9 10 03 02 01 00 99 98 97 96 95 94

God Gave Me My Sense of Taste

Lemons taste sour and pepper tastes hot.
Pickles taste salty, but apples do not.
Real chocolate is bitter, so not good to eat . . .
Unless sugar's added . . . and then it tastes sweet!
I'm sure there are flavors we favor among
All of God's gifts which we taste with our tongue!

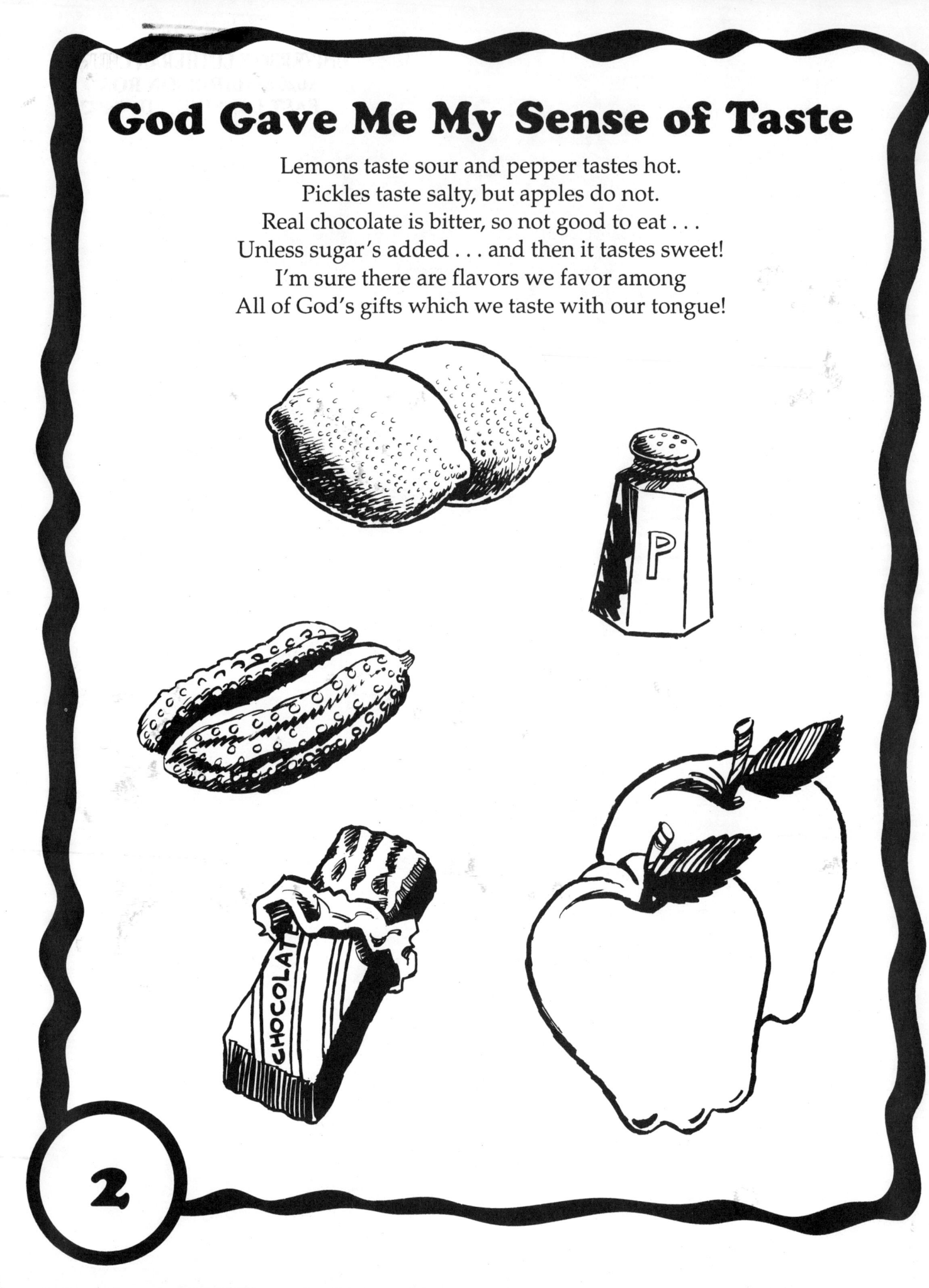

2

A Thank-You Place Mat

1. Write a thank-You prayer to God on a piece of construction paper. Thank Him for giving you good food to eat.

2. Draw pictures of your favorite foods around your prayer.

3. Ask a grown-up to help you cut slits all around the edge of the paper to make fringe.

4. If you wish, cover the place mat with clear adhesive paper.

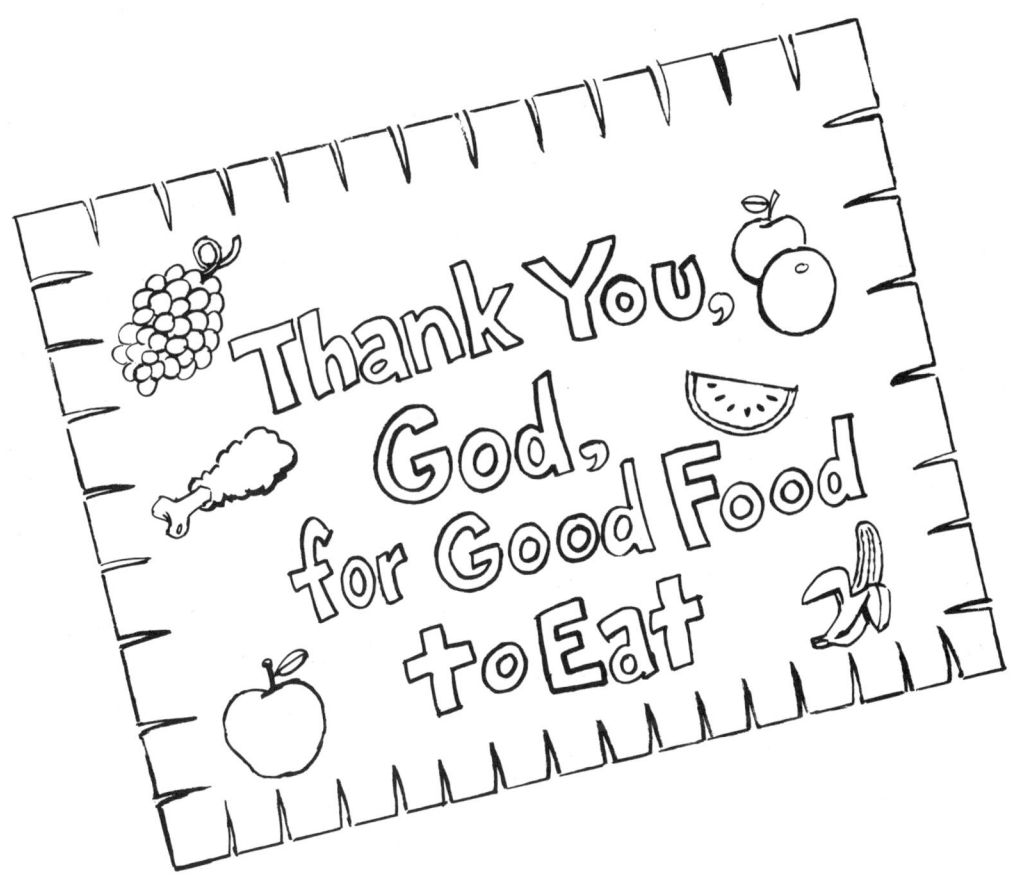

In Bible times people used honey instead of sugar to sweeten their food. Connect the dots to find a sweet treat we enjoy today.

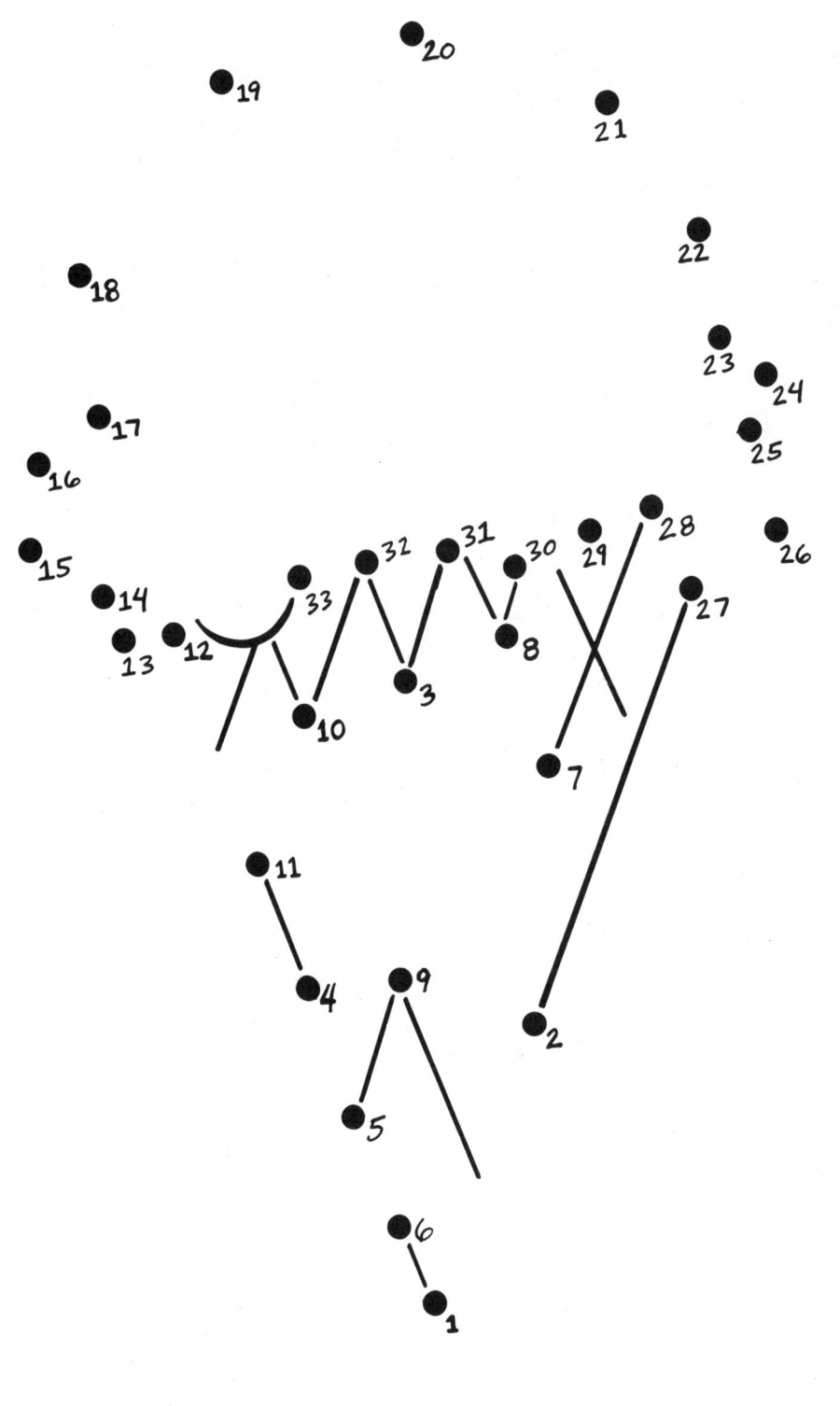

The names of 10 kinds of fruit are hidden in these sentences. The first one is found for you. Can you find the rest?

1. We could be shepherds <u>or angels</u> in the Christmas play.
2. Always ask God to help you figure out your problems.
3. We will never stop praising God for His blessings.
4. Dad built my tree house out of scrap lumber.
5. Mom wrapped a lot of tape around the box.
6. I did every problem on the chalkboard.
7. I like the taste of melon on ice cream.
8. God tells us to help each other.
9. My puppy can do lively tricks.
10. I meet a new friend at each Sunday school class.

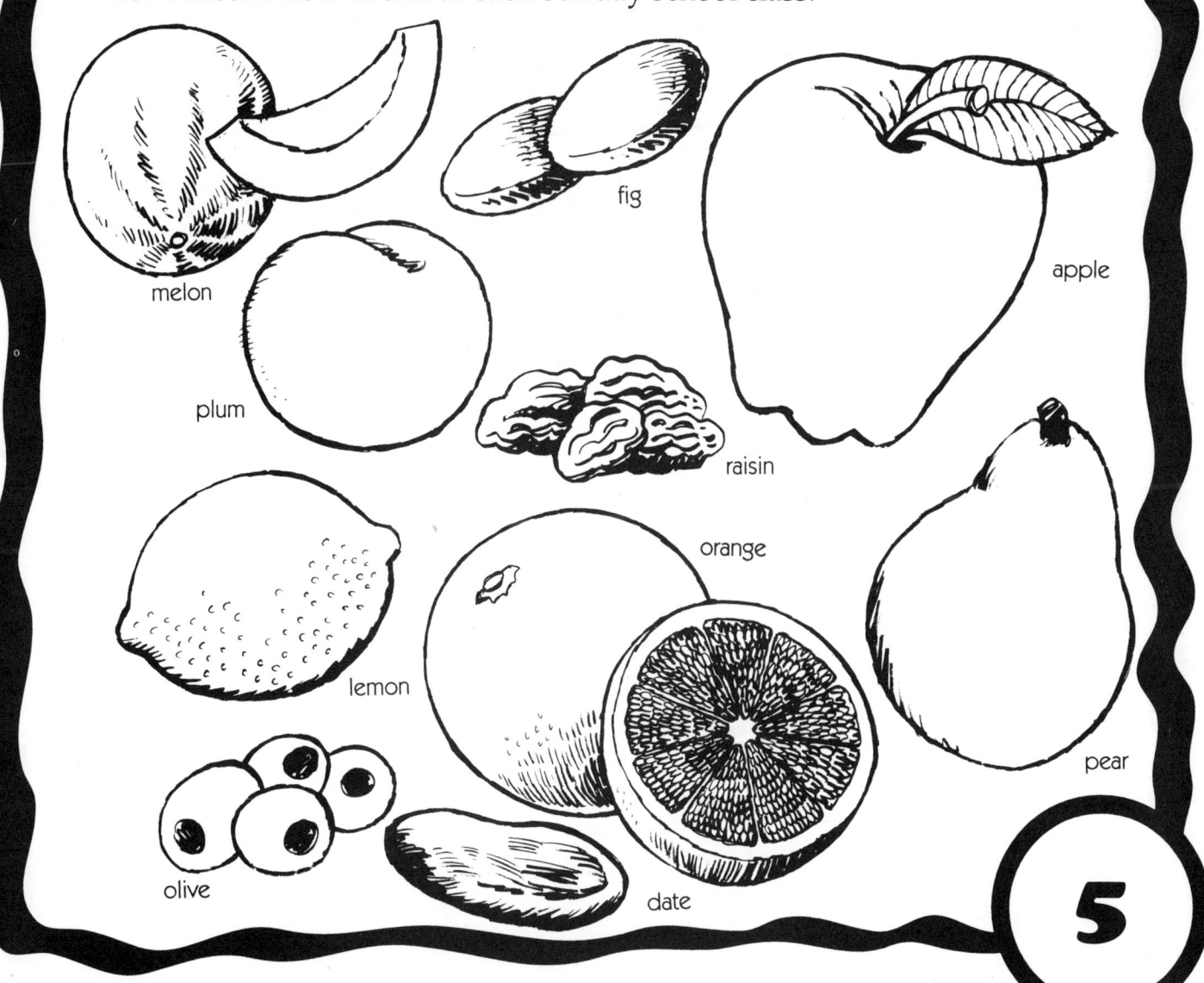

Make Your Favorite Meal

1. Cut out pictures of your favorite foods from magazines.
2. Glue the pictures on a paper plate to make a meal.

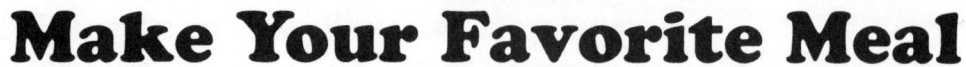

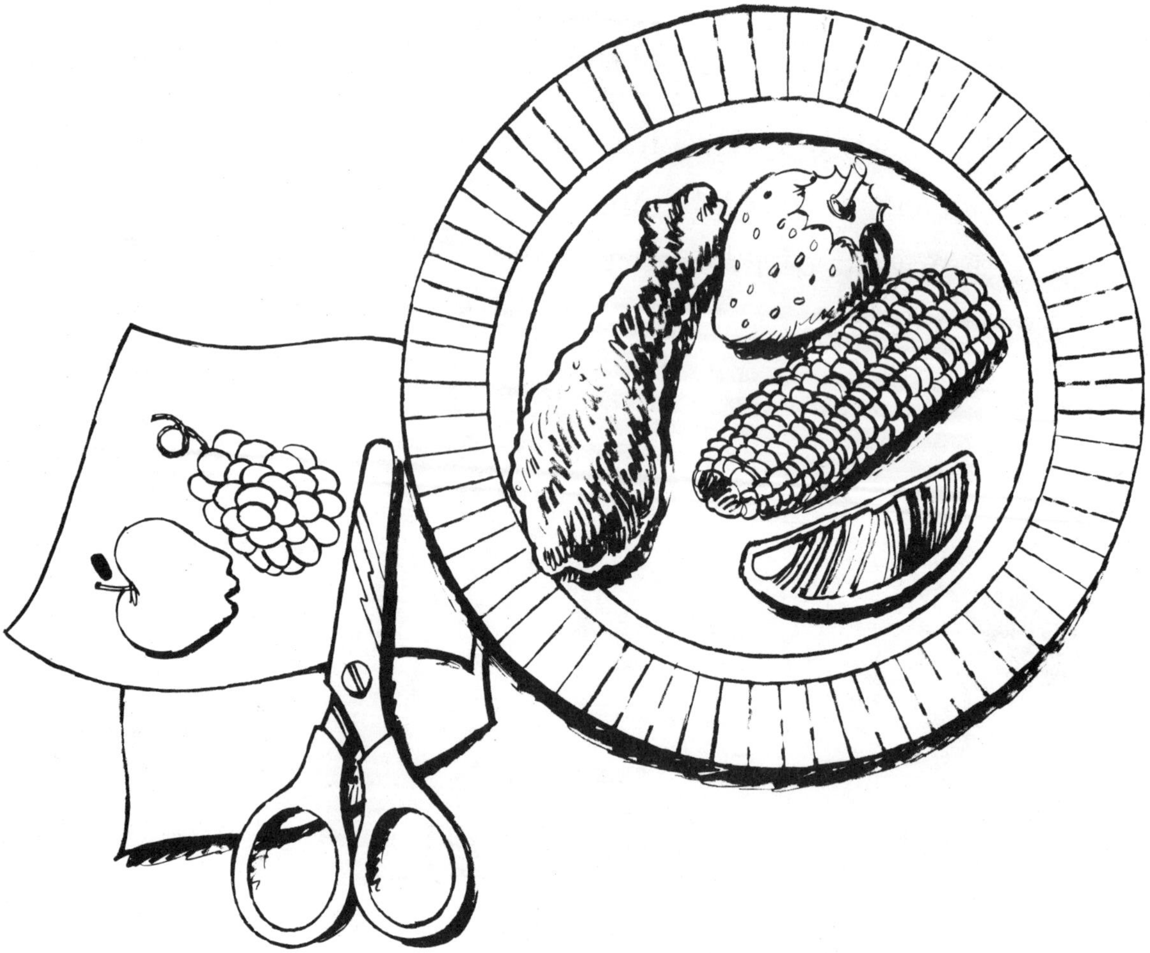

In Old Testament times David took care of his father's sheep. He took food with him to the pasture so he wouldn't get hungry. Find and circle the following words in the word puzzle. Words are printed across and down.

GRAPES DATES CHEESE OLIVES
HONEY BREAD FIGS RAISINS

G	R	A	P	E	S	A	D	A	T	E	S	E
M	P	Z	I	Q	W	N	R	T	O	I	Y	R
G	H	B	B	D	K	R	V	J	F	C	M	A
Q	W	R	E	R	T	Y	U	I	F	O	P	I
C	H	E	E	S	E	A	O	L	I	V	E	S
S	D	A	S	F	G	H	J	K	G	L	Z	I
X	C	D	V	B	N	M	Q	W	S	E	R	N
T	Y	U	F	H	O	N	E	Y	H	O	D	S

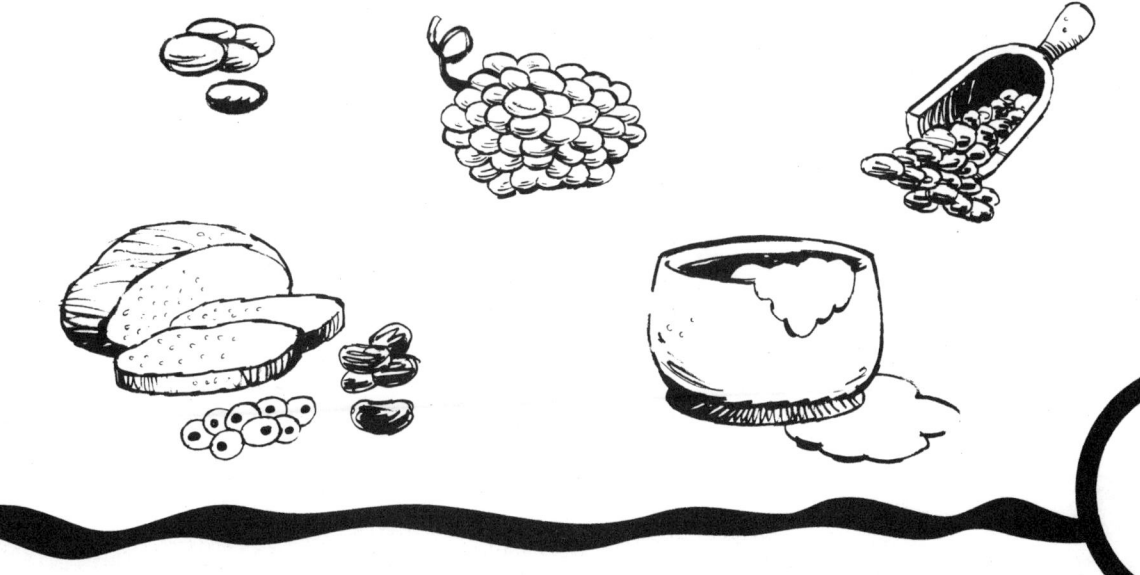

7

Fudgy Frozen Treats

Ingredients

3 ½ cups milk
1   3½-oz. chocolate pudding mix (not instant)
1 egg, beaten

Directions

1. Stir milk and pudding mix until smooth.

2. Ask a grown-up to help you place in microwave (high), uncovered, for 10 to 12 minutes, until mixture boils and thickens. Stir 2 or 3 times while heating.

3. Blend half of chocolate mixture with beaten egg; then return to pudding mixture and stir until smooth.

4. Microwave (high), uncovered, 1 to 1 ½ minutes, until edges bubble. Cool, stirring occasionally.

5. Divide mixture into paper cups. Insert a plastic spoon into center of each. Freeze until firm, about 6 hours.

6. To serve, peel off paper and enjoy. (If treats are frozen too hard, microwave for 10 seconds. Then twist out of cup.)

More Ideas

1. Use different flavors of pudding.
2. Use plastic frozen treat molds instead of paper cups.

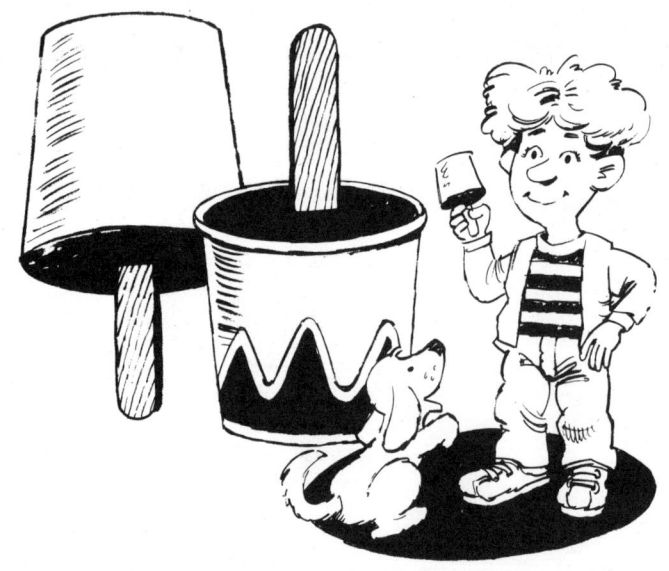

God Gave Me My Sense of Sight

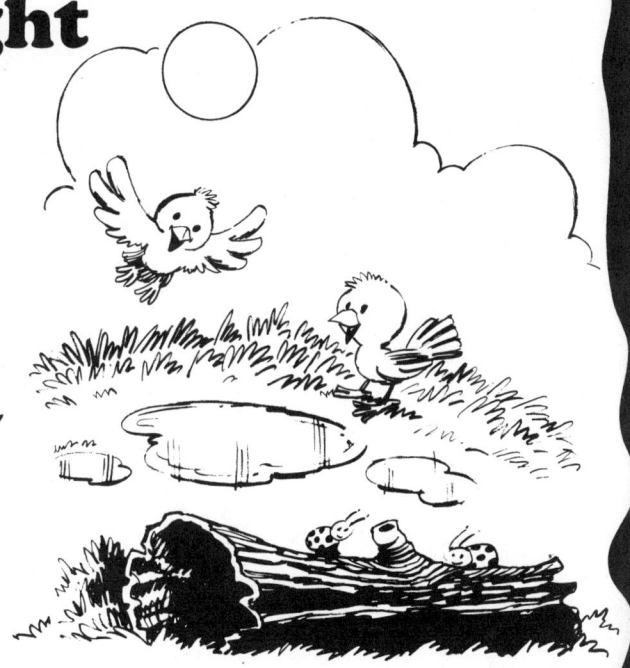

God gave us sight so we might see
The gifts He made for you and me!
When we look *up*, we see the sky,
And many different birds that fly.
God made the daytime clouds so white,
And then the sparkling stars at night.
When we look *down*, we see green grass,
Or pools of rain that look like glass.
If we're inside, we might see rugs,
Or outside, maybe ladybugs.
How wonderful it is to see
All things God made for you and me!

God made many gifts for you to enjoy. Write some of His gifts that you can see right now.

When I look up, I see _____.

When I look down, I see _____.

When I look straight ahead, I see _____.

When I look through a window, I see _____.

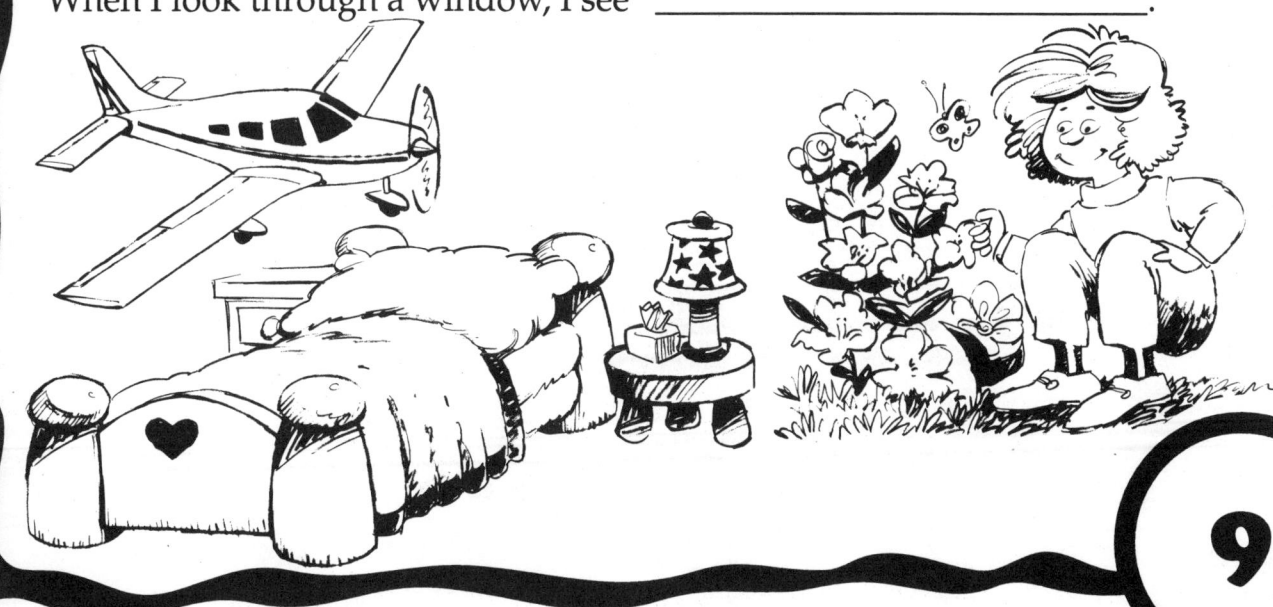

9

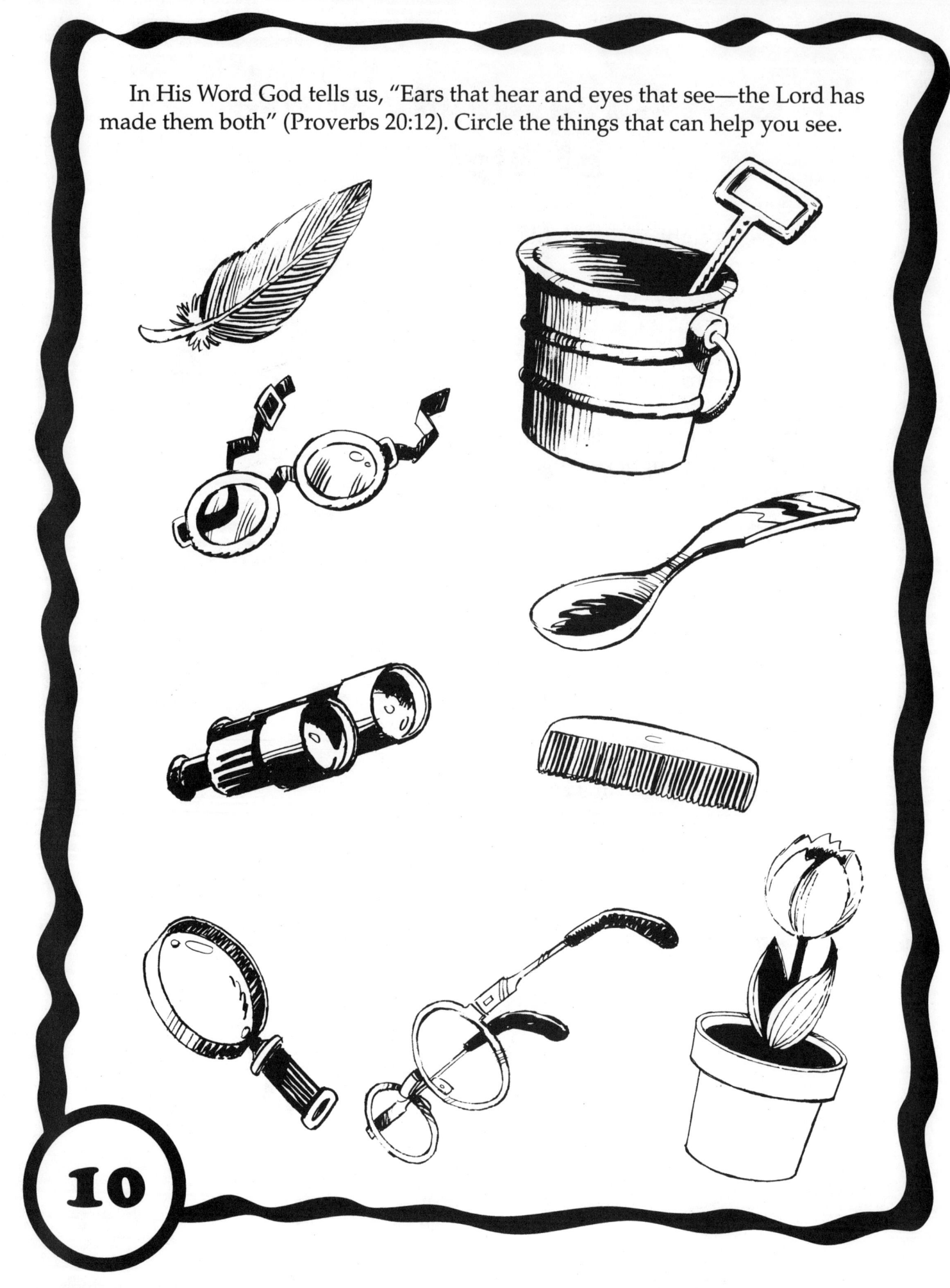

Color the Rainbow

Noah and his family saw a beautiful rainbow in the sky after the great flood. God placed the rainbow in the sky as a promise that He would never again destroy the entire earth with a flood. Match the numbers to color the rainbow.

1 red
2 orange
3 yellow
4 green
5 blue
6 indigo
7 violet

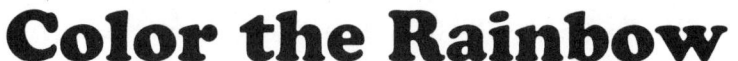

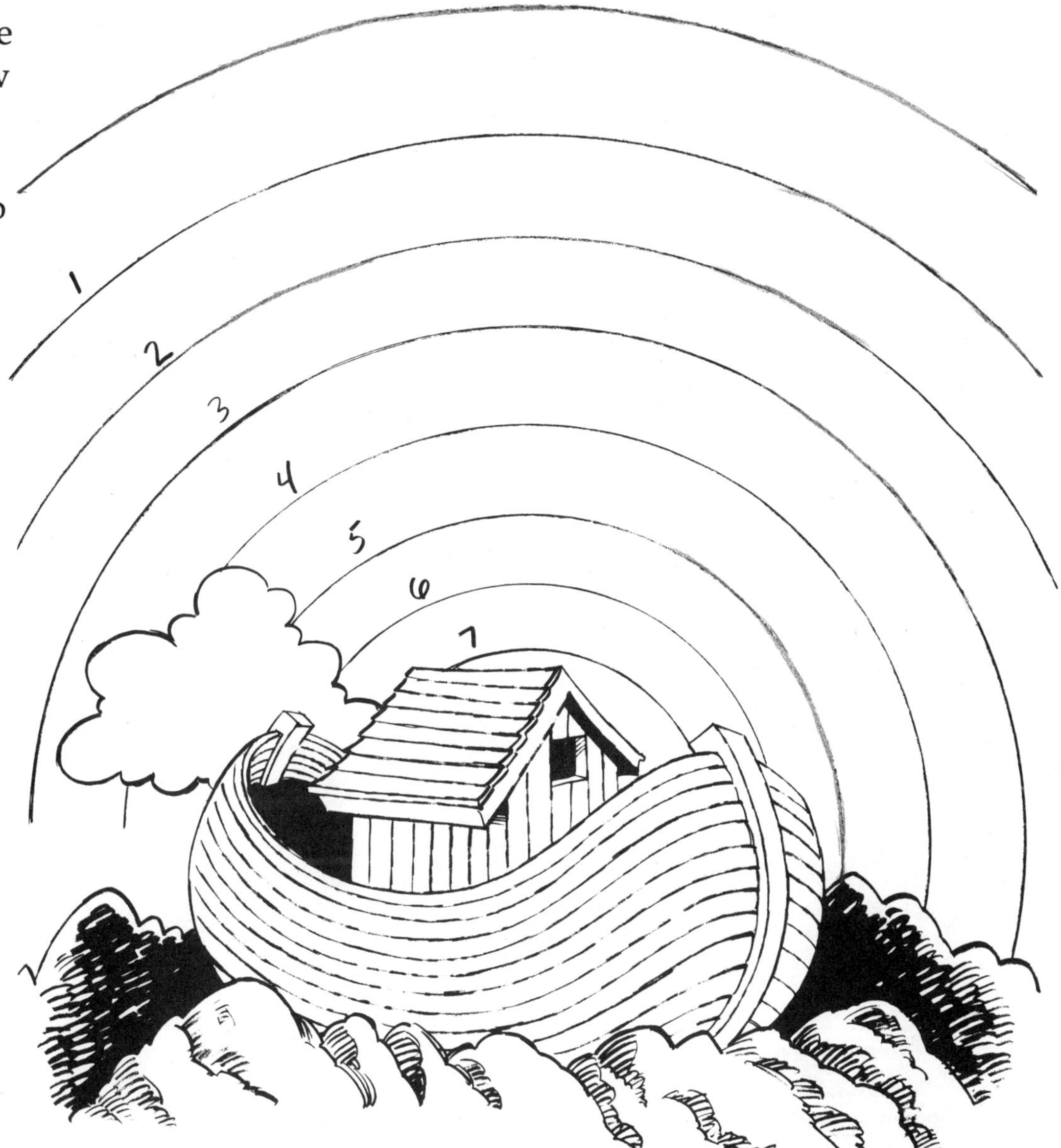

God's children saw many things on their journey from Egypt to the Promised Land of Canaan. Solve the crossword puzzle to learn about some of these things.

Word Box

SEA   MOUNTAINS
FIRE   SAND
ROCK   QUAIL
CLOUD

Across

4. A bright _ _ _ _ _ guided them by day.
5. They traveled over hot _ _ _ _ .
6. A pillar of _ _ _ _ led them by night.

Down

1. They saw Moses strike a _ _ _ _ with his rod to get water.
2. They saw some tall _ _ _ _ _ _ _ _ _ .
3. They were surprised to see _ _ _ _ _ in the desert. (God sent these birds to the Israelites when they were hungry and could not find food.)
5. They escaped Pharaoh's army by crossing the Red _ _ _ on a path of dry ground.

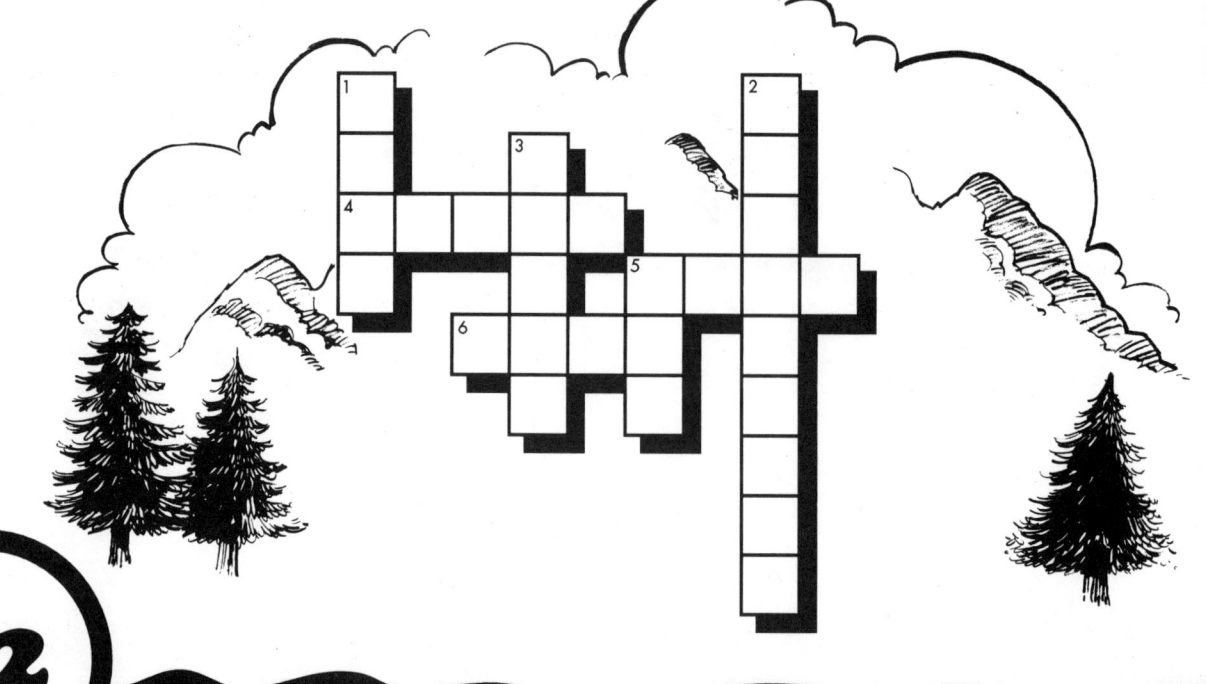

12

God makes different kinds of eyes. Some can see and some cannot. Circle the things that have eyes and *can* see. Draw a line under the things that have eyes but *cannot* see.

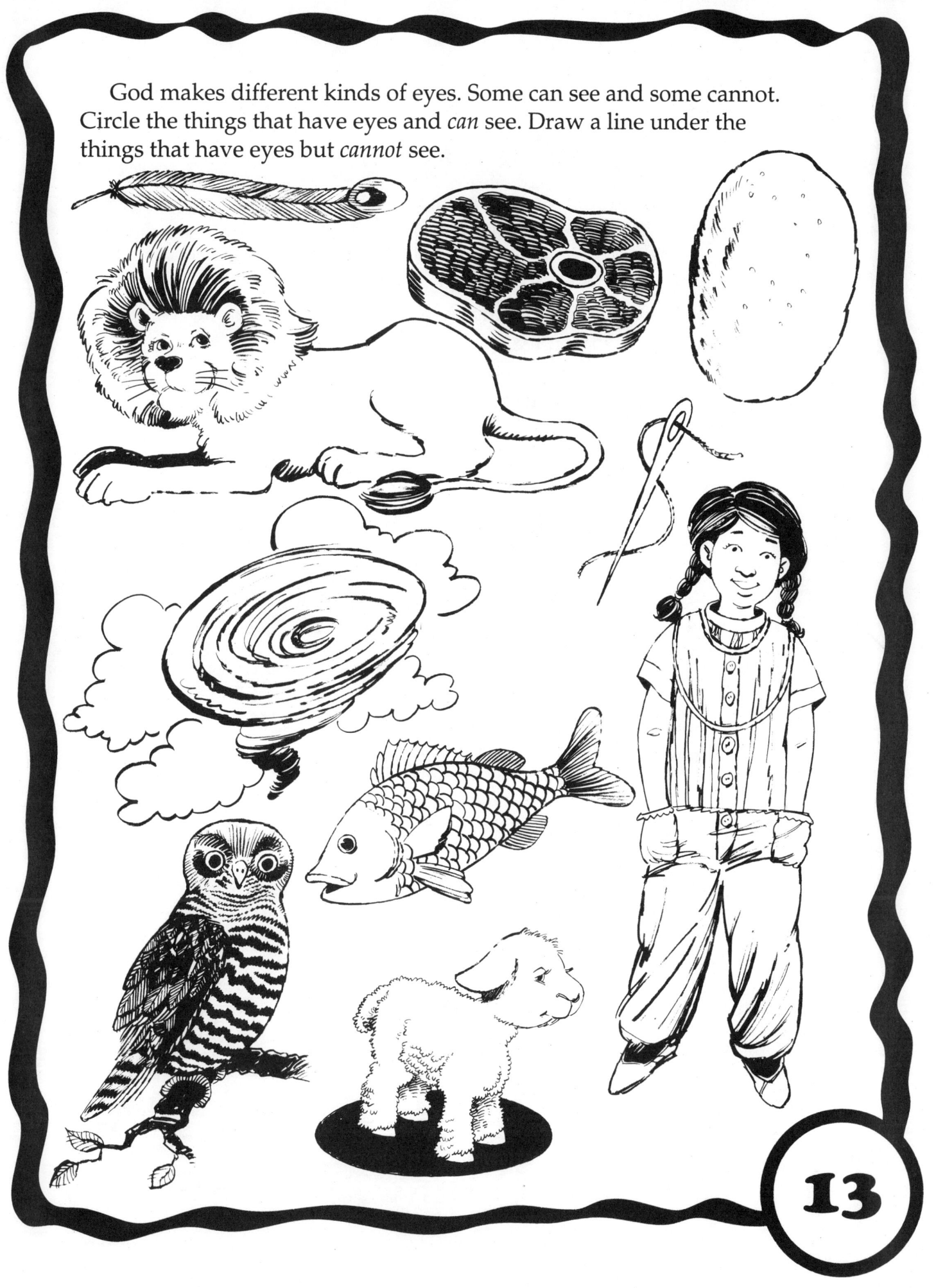

God Gave Me My Sense of Touch

Have you ever squeezed a marshmallow?
    It's like a fluffy pillow.
Have you ever felt the silky fur
    Of a pussy willow?
Now, following a nice, warm bath,
    Do you feel warm and rosy,
Especially when you're tucked beneath
    Your blanket, warm and cozy?
Have you ever licked a Popsicle
    Or ice cream on a stick?
I'm sure your tongue felt colder with
    Each tummy-tempting lick!
God gives us all good gifts because
    He loves us, oh, so much!
I'm glad He blessed us with this gift . . .
    The gift to feel and touch!

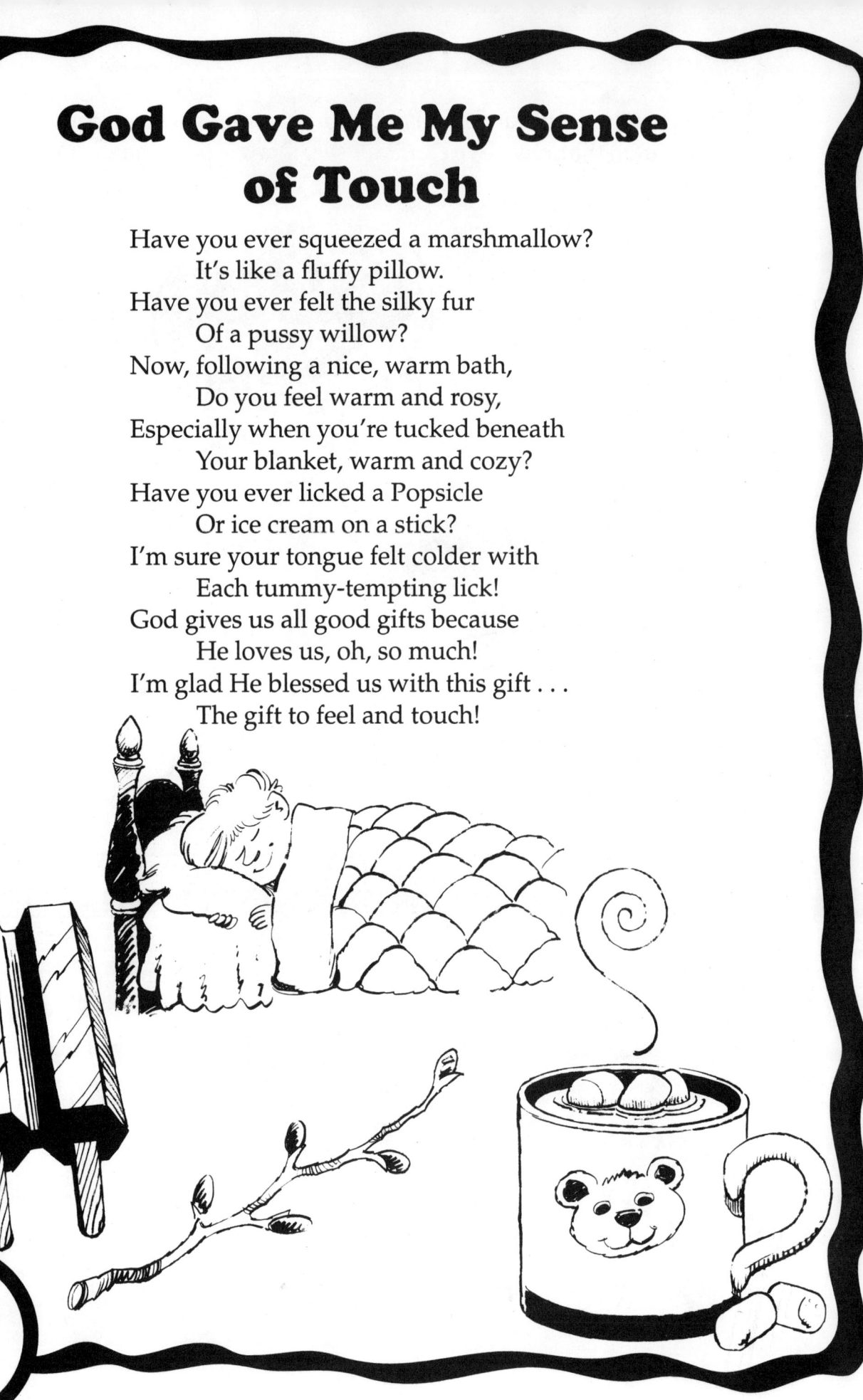

In the spring it feels good to dig your hands into warm, moist earth. You can plant seeds and enjoy God's gifts of flowers and plants.

A Garden in Egg Shells

Whenever Mother breaks an egg,
   Be sure to save the shell;
Then fill each half with soil and seed—
   Be sure to water well.
When you have finished planting, then
   Replace them in the carton;
Come spring you'll have green, growing sprouts
   To transplant in your garden!

Tips

1. Remove top of egg carton.

2. Follow directions on seed package for planting time.

3. Place carton on a sunny windowsill.

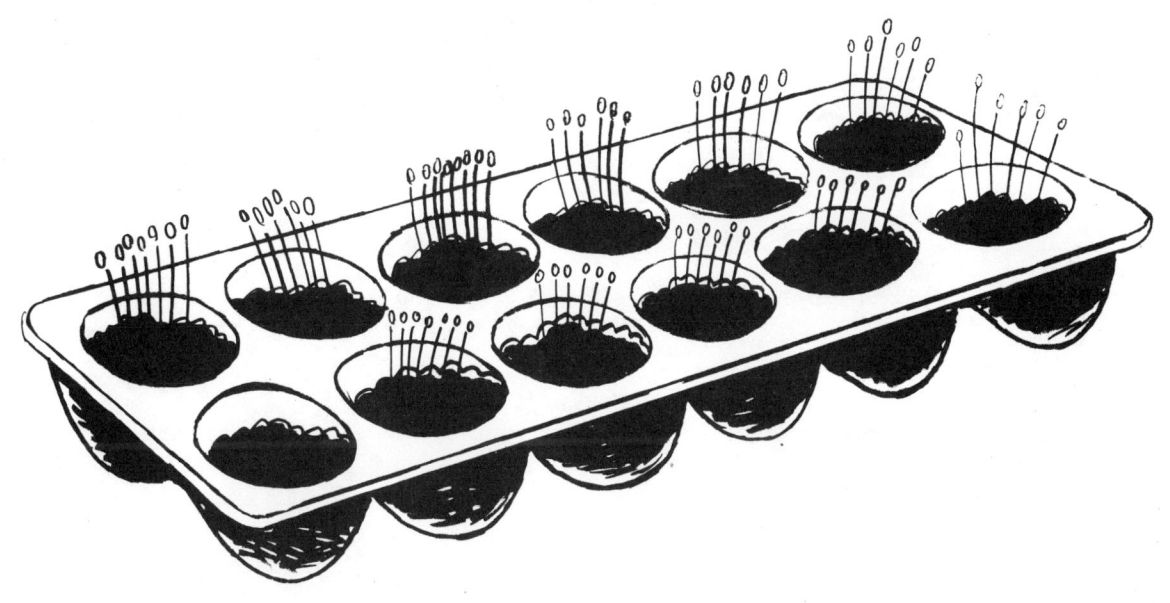

When you play outside in the winter, you wear a warm jacket or snowsuit. In the summer you might wear shorts or a swimsuit. Animals feel the heat and cold just like we do. But animals do not have clothes to put on or take off like we do.

God was very wise when He planned places for His animals to live. Some animals live in places where it is always hot. Some live in places where it is always cold. Use a *red* crayon to circle animals that like *hot* weather. Use a *blue* crayon to circle animals that like *cold* weather.

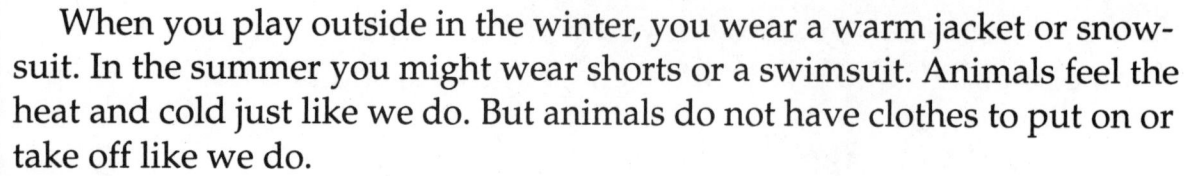

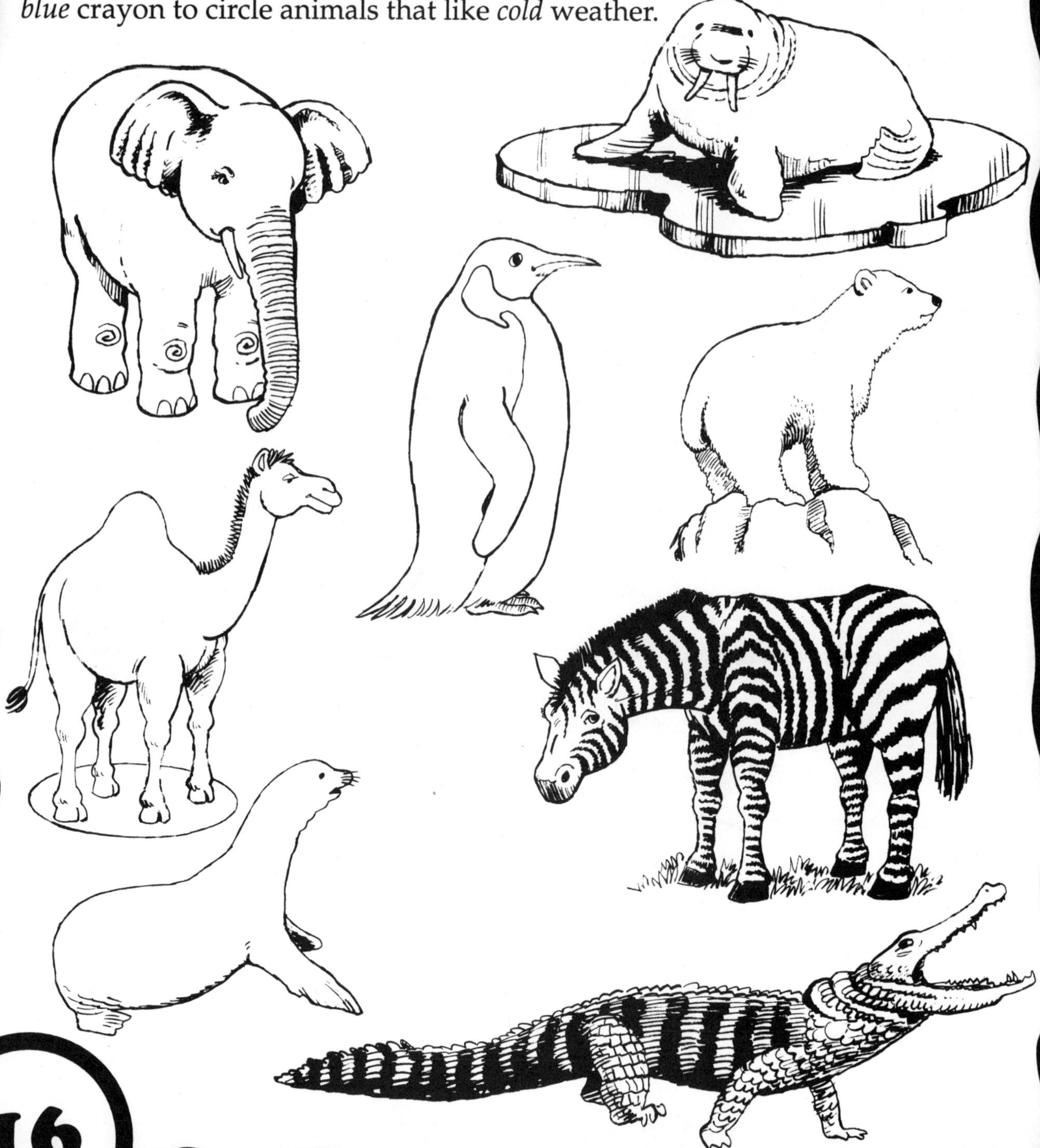

Pictures You Can Touch and Feel

You can make pictures from bark that is prickly;
Then add leaves and feathers so it will feel tickly.
Some things could be knobby, like nuts, and feel lumpy;
Then add seeds and twigs so your picture is bumpy.
Some pieces of fabric will make it feel patchy,
And surely some beach sand will make it feel scratchy.

You can find things to make a touch-and-feel picture in many places—the park, in the woods, by a river, at the beach, even in your own backyard.

Put the things you find on a sheet of cardboard. Move them around until they make a design or picture that you like. Then glue or tape them in place.

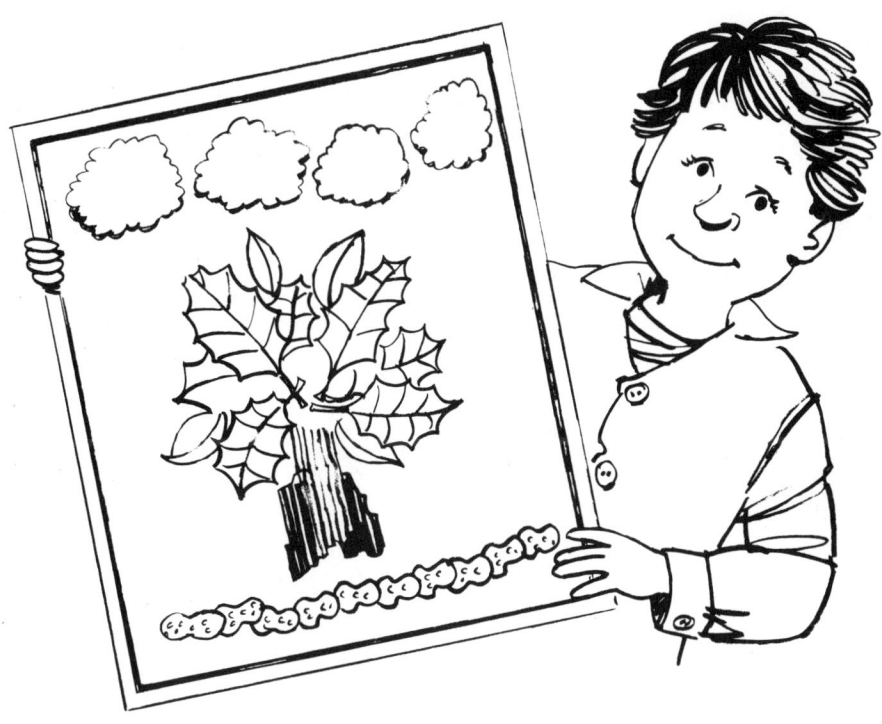

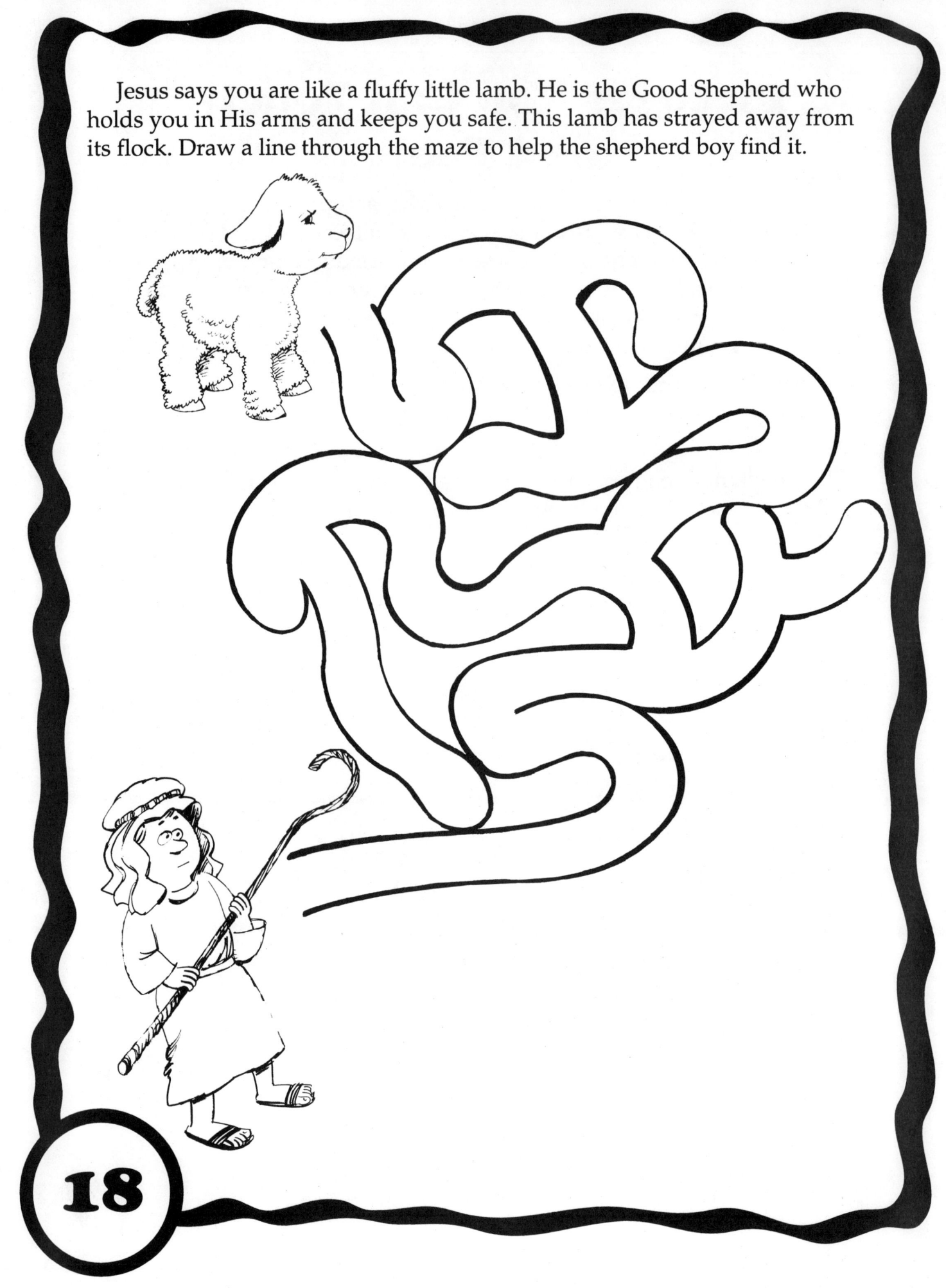

It is fun to feel different things in God's world. Draw a line from the objects on the left to the word on the right that describes how they feel.

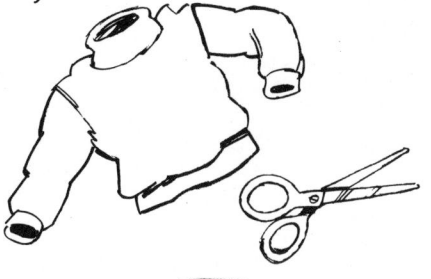

shaggy

furry

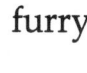

crunchy

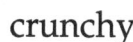

rough

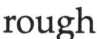

warm

sharp

gooey

scratchy

hard

soft

tickly

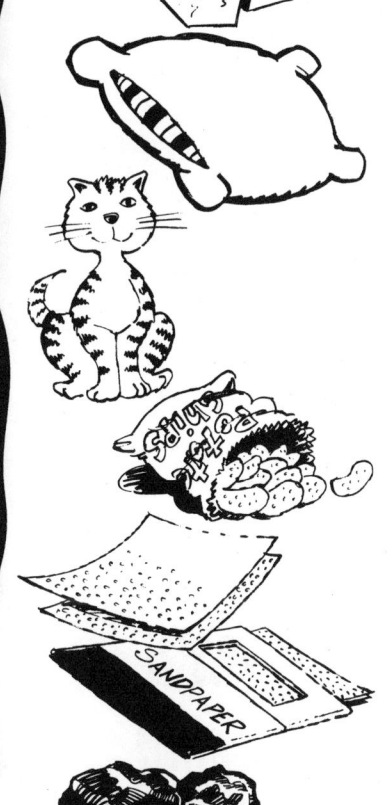

God Gave Me My Sense of Smell

God wanted us to smell His world,
    That's why He gave us noses!
Just think of all the things we smell
    From apple pie to roses!
When mother bakes a loaf of bread,
    Just take a great big whiff,
And when it comes to peppermint,
    Can you resist a sniff?
With eyes closed you could play a game—
    You easily could tell
What's right beneath your nose because
    You have the sense of smell!

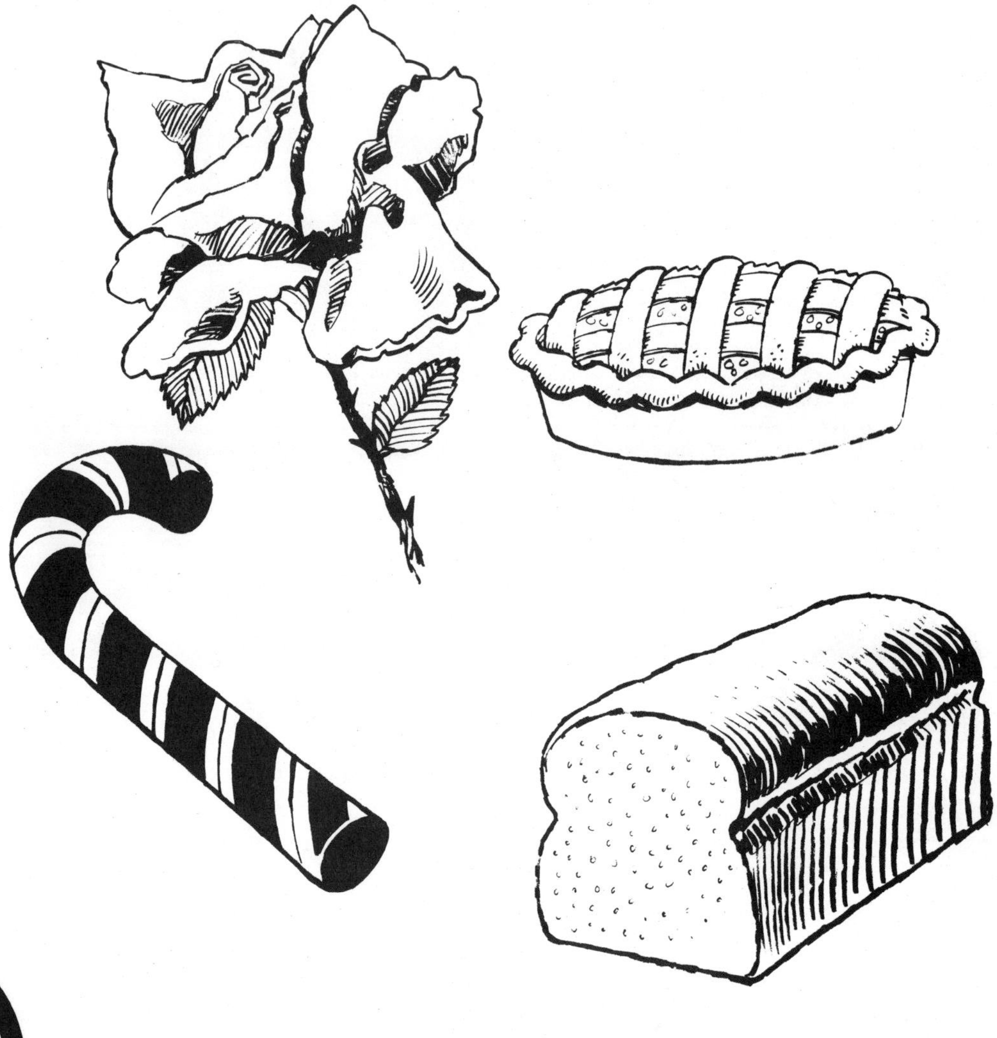

God gives us beautiful flowers to smell. In each row, circle the two flowers that are alike.

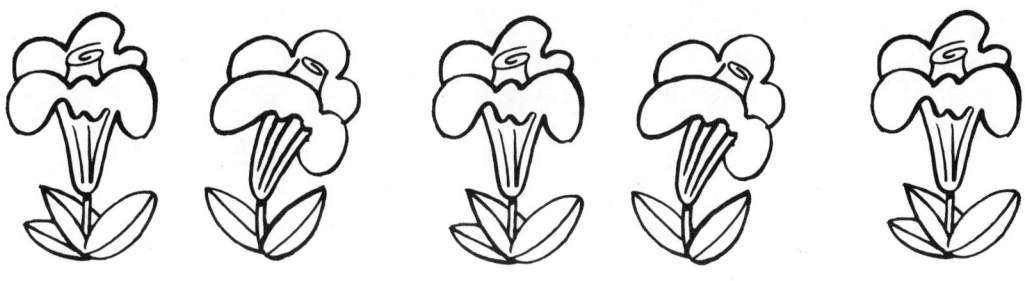

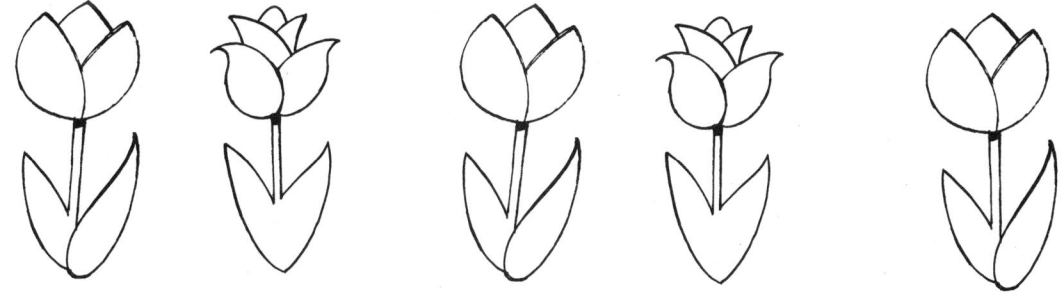

Sailboat Salad

Like many fruits that God made, peaches have a nice smell. You can make a sailboat salad that will look good and smell great!

1. Rinse a lettuce leaf and lay it on a plate.

2. Ask a grown-up to help you open a can of peaches. Place a peach half on the lettuce, rounded side down.

3. Cut a small sail from paper.

4. Stick a toothpick through the paper to make a mast. Stick the end of the toothpick into the peach. (If you have a party, you could print the name of each of your guests on a sail. Then your salads would also be place cards.)

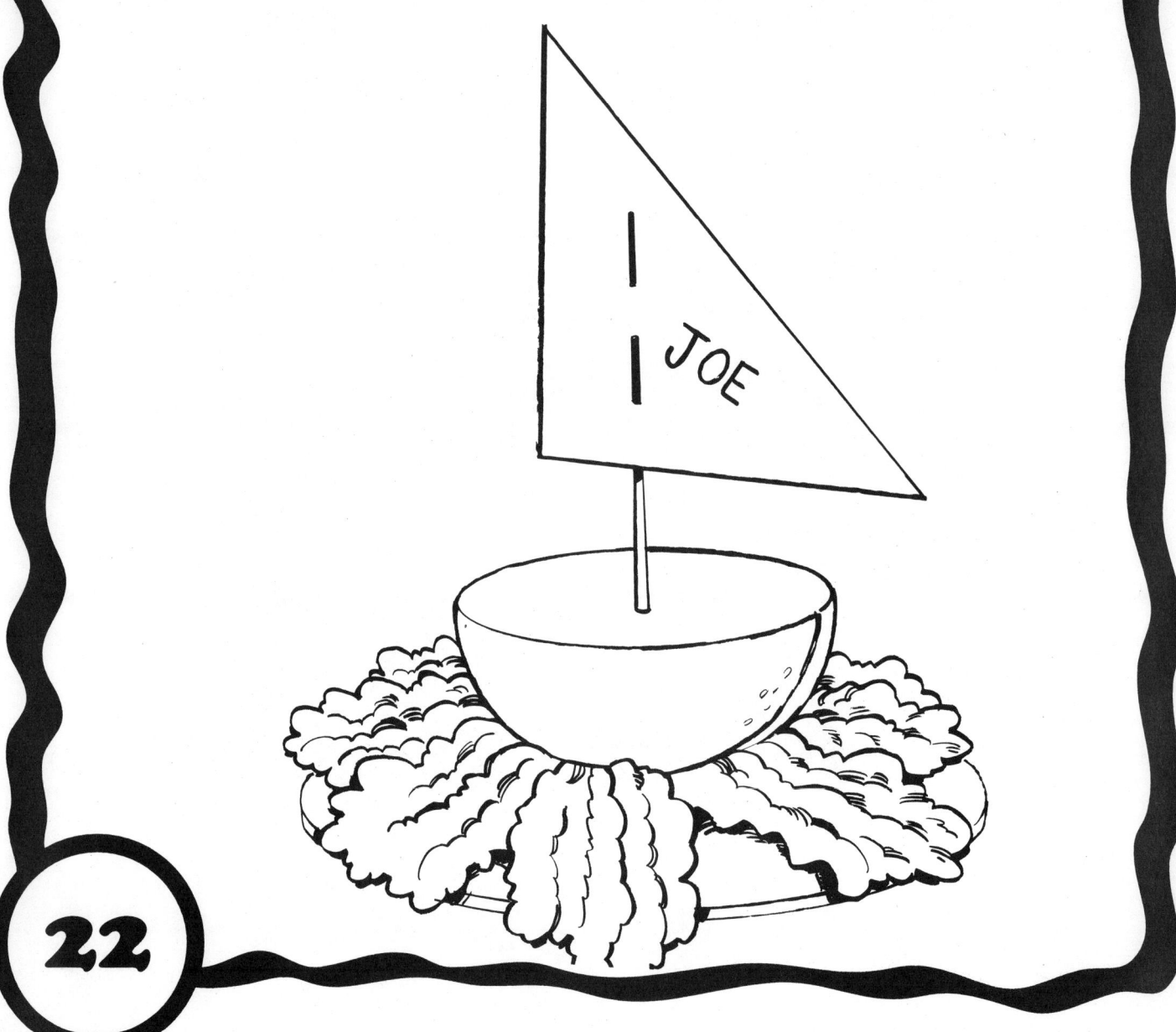

In the summer we smell fresh, new grass,
In winter, cold, crisp air.
Let's not forget God's gifts to us,
But say a thank-You prayer!

With a *blue* crayon, circle the things you might smell in the *winter*.
With a *green* crayon, circle the things you might smell in the *summer*.

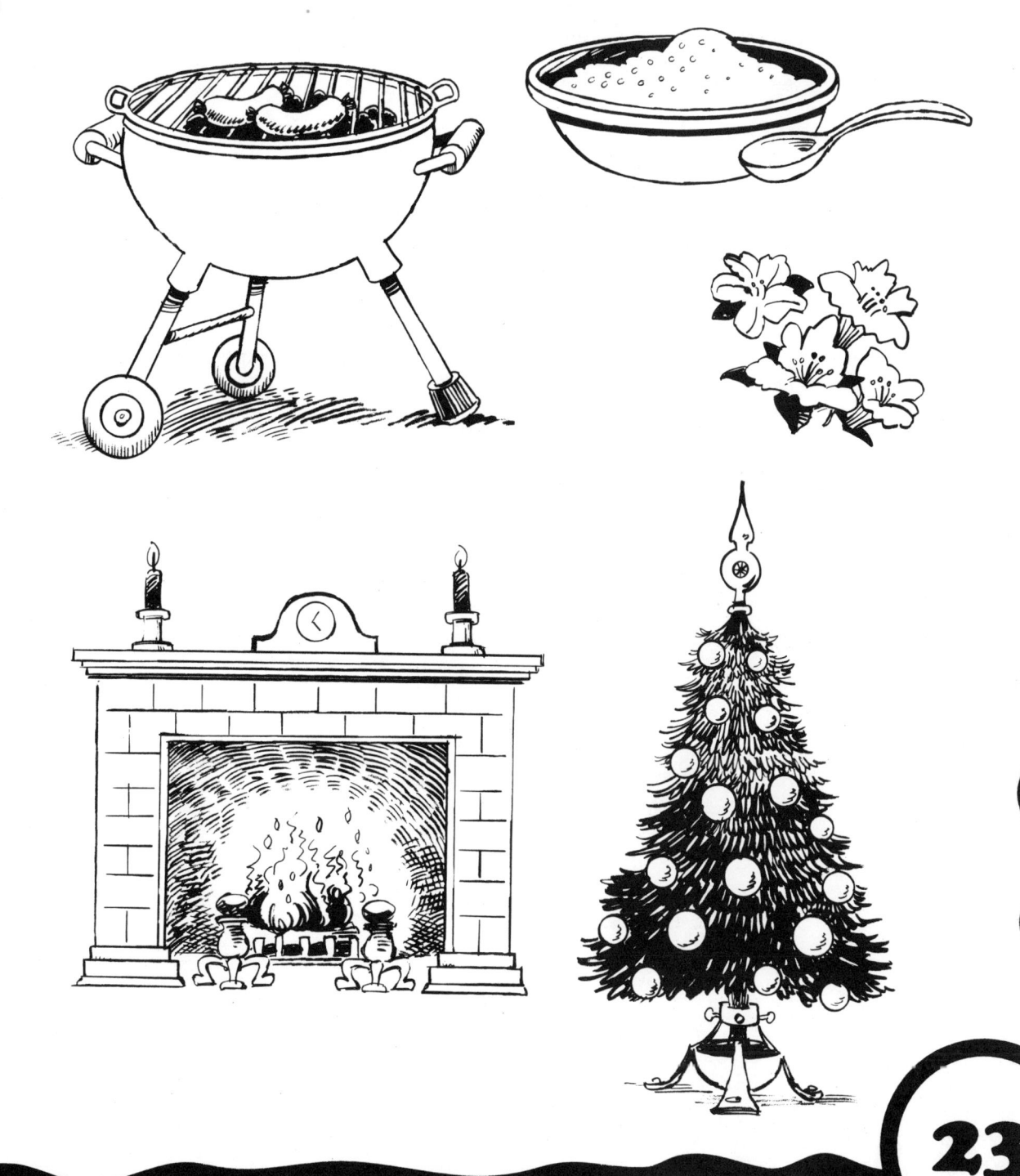

What Is Wrong with This Picture?

There are six things in the picture that should not have noses. Can you find them? Aren't you glad that God gave you a nose?

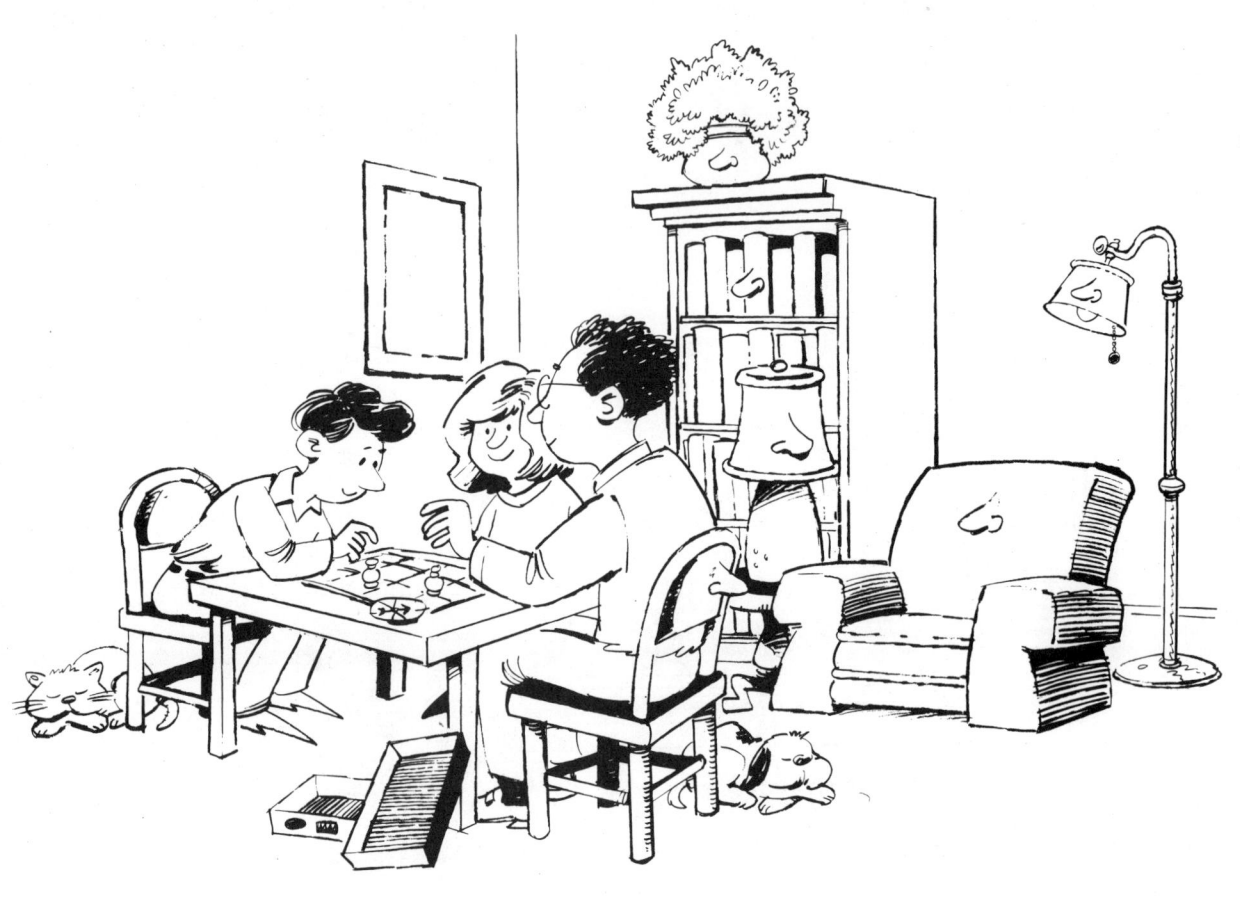

24

Nosy Bookmarks

Copy this page. Color the clowns and carefully cut on the dotted lines. Slip a clown's nose over a page you want to mark in a book. God makes noses in many shapes and sizes!

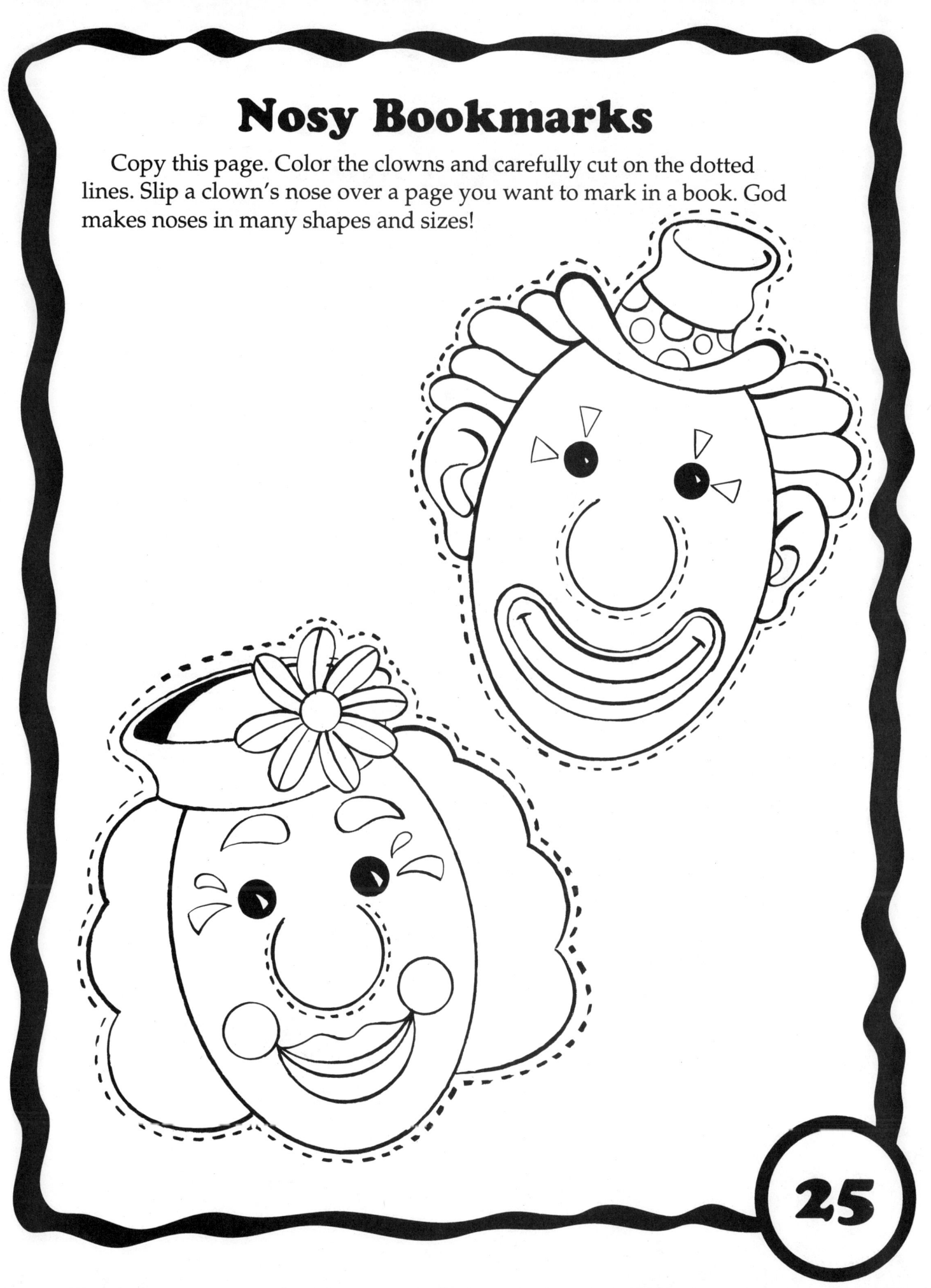

25

God Gave Me My Sense of Hearing

I'm glad God gave me ears to hear
    The croaks of Mr. Frog;
The soft meows from Puff, my cat;
    And barks from Sam, my dog.
I can hear the thunder crash,
    Or gentle rain that falls,
And when I'm playing I can hear
    My mother when she calls.
I'm glad God gave me ears to hear
    So many things each day.
I'm even happier to know
    God hears me when I pray!

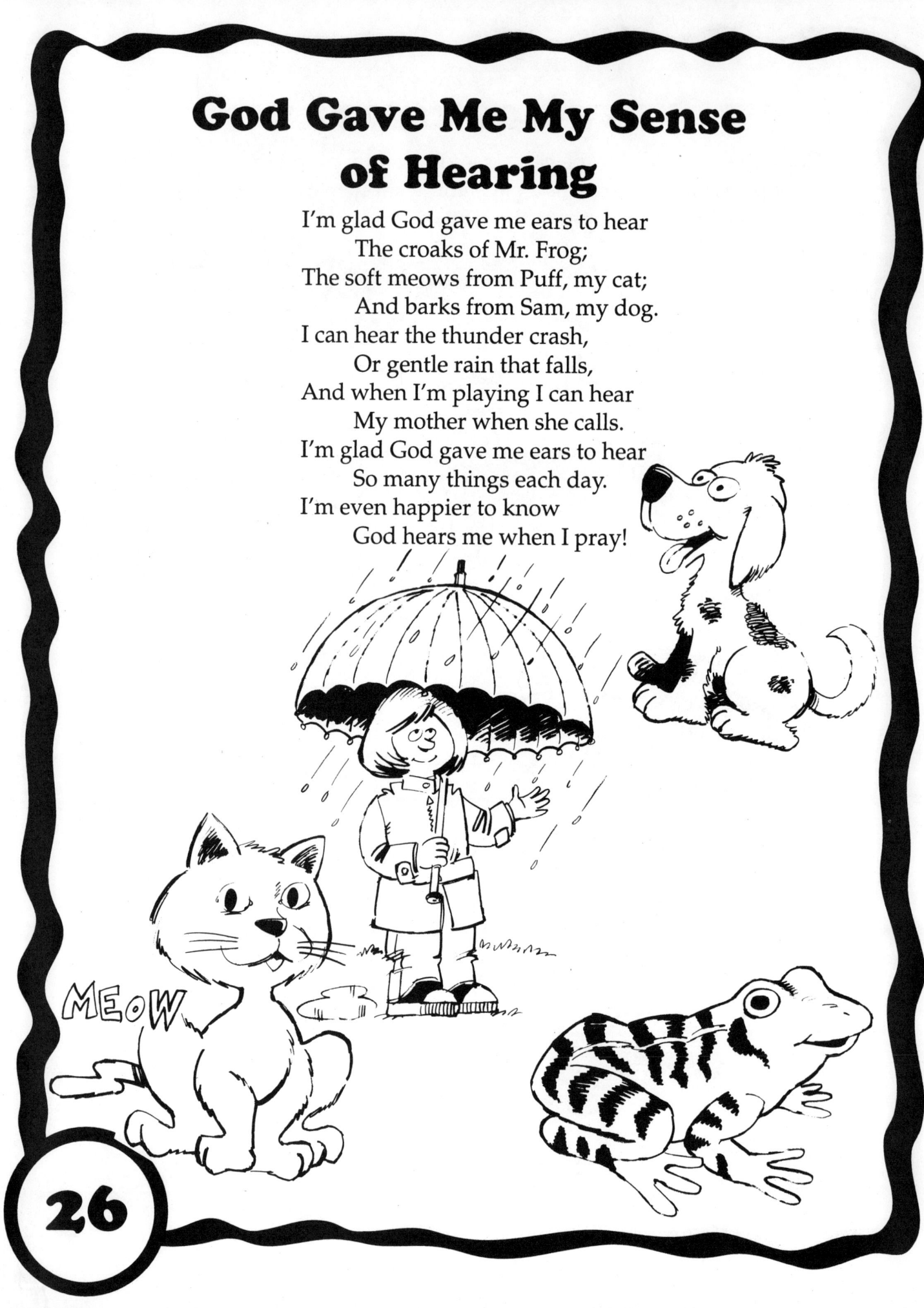

These people are missing their ears! Draw ears for them so they can hear.

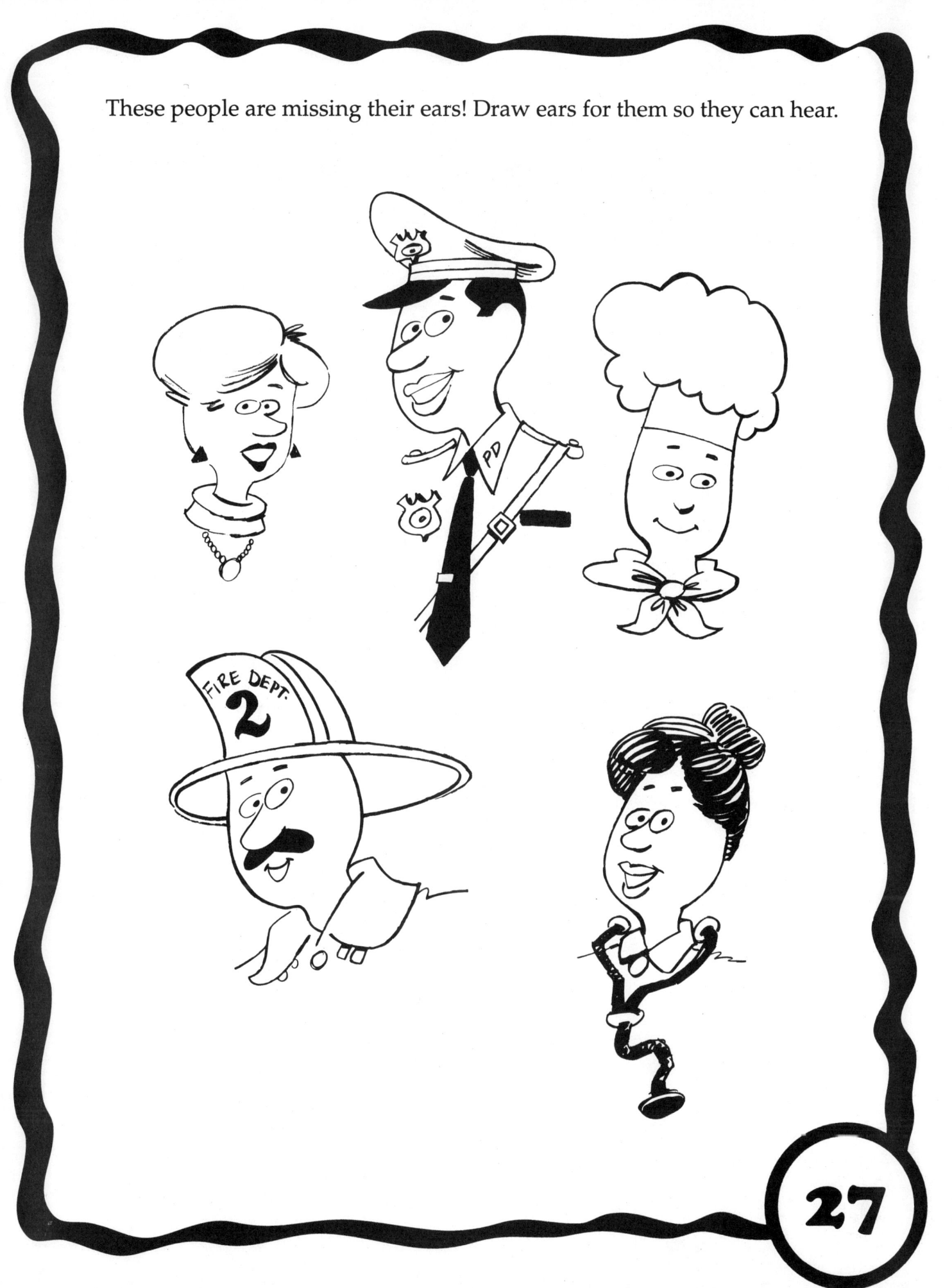

27

When you hold this object to your ear, you will hear a sound like the ocean. Connect the dots to find out what it is.

When God created the earth, He made strange and wonderful creatures to live in the ocean.

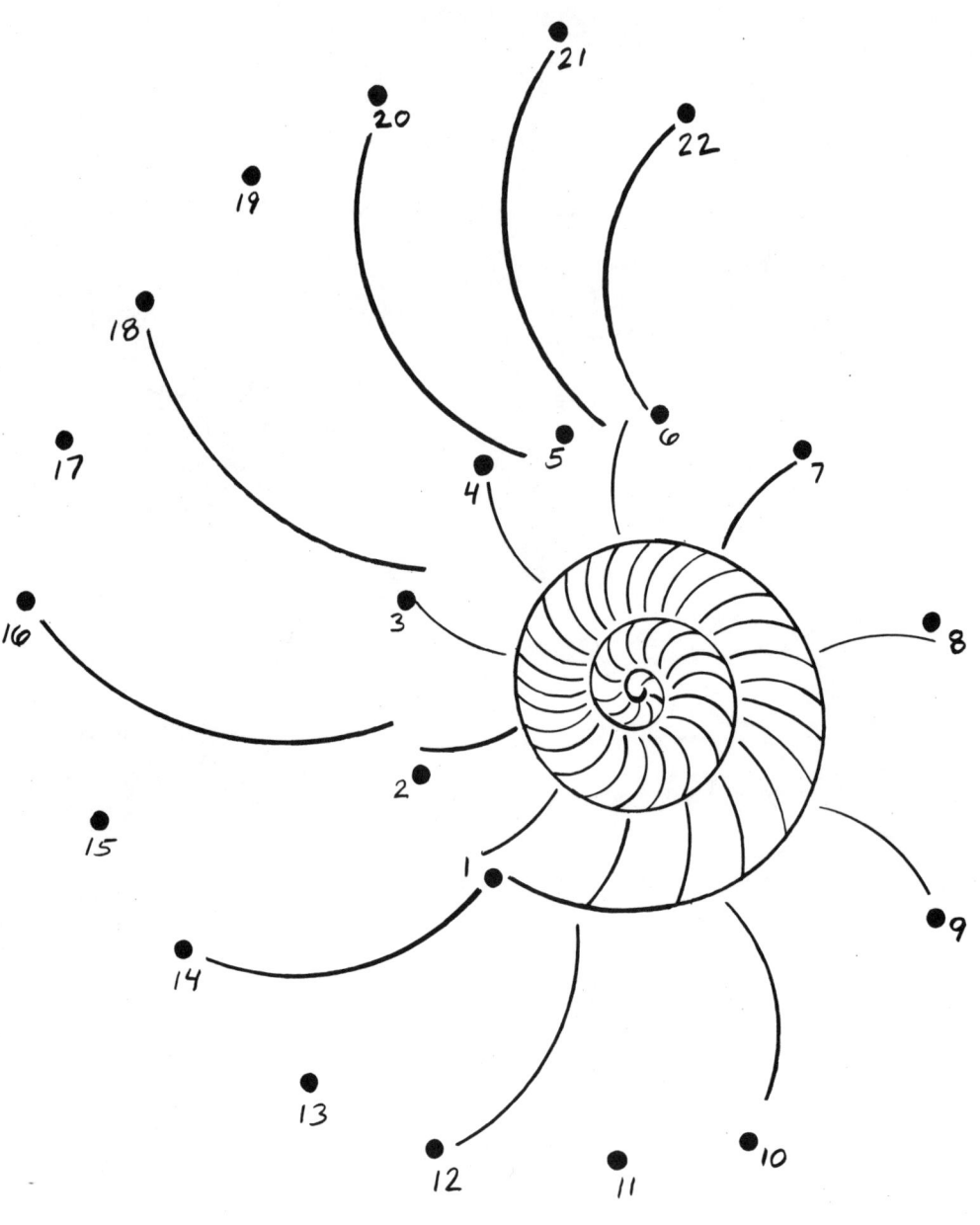

28

Praise God with Music

Drum 'n' Strum Some Musical Fun

A comb and waxed paper will make a fine flute.
A tube made of cardboard? A horn you can toot!
A can for a drum with a stick to *bang, bang,*
And rubber bands stretched on a board will *twang, twang.*
Line up on the sidewalk, then march to the beat . . .
And surely you'll be the best band on your street.

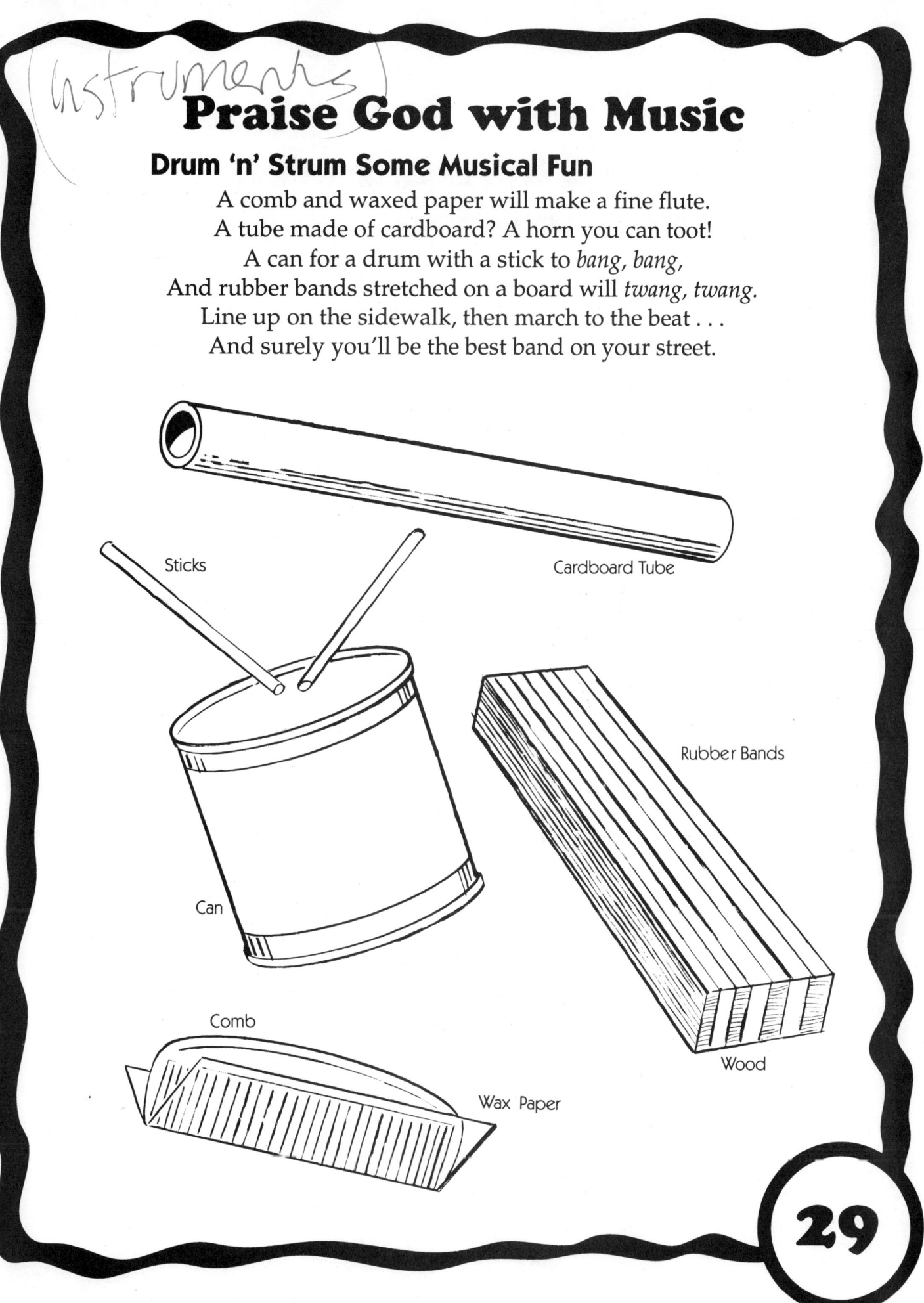

Help the Animals Find Their Ears

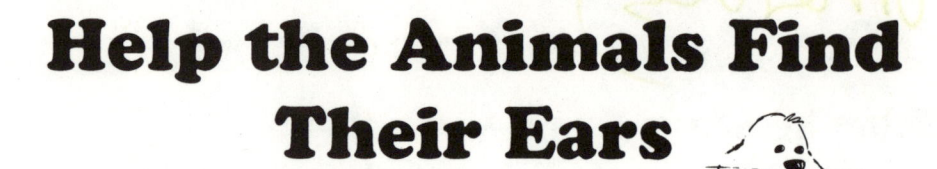

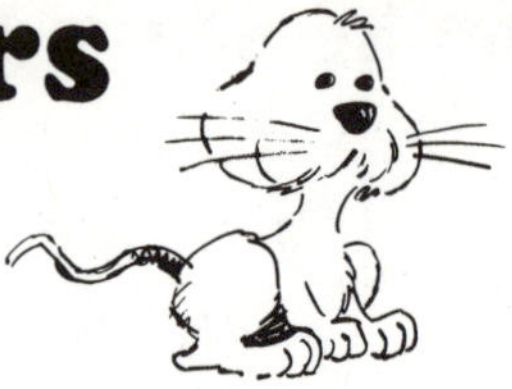

Draw a line from each animal to its ears.

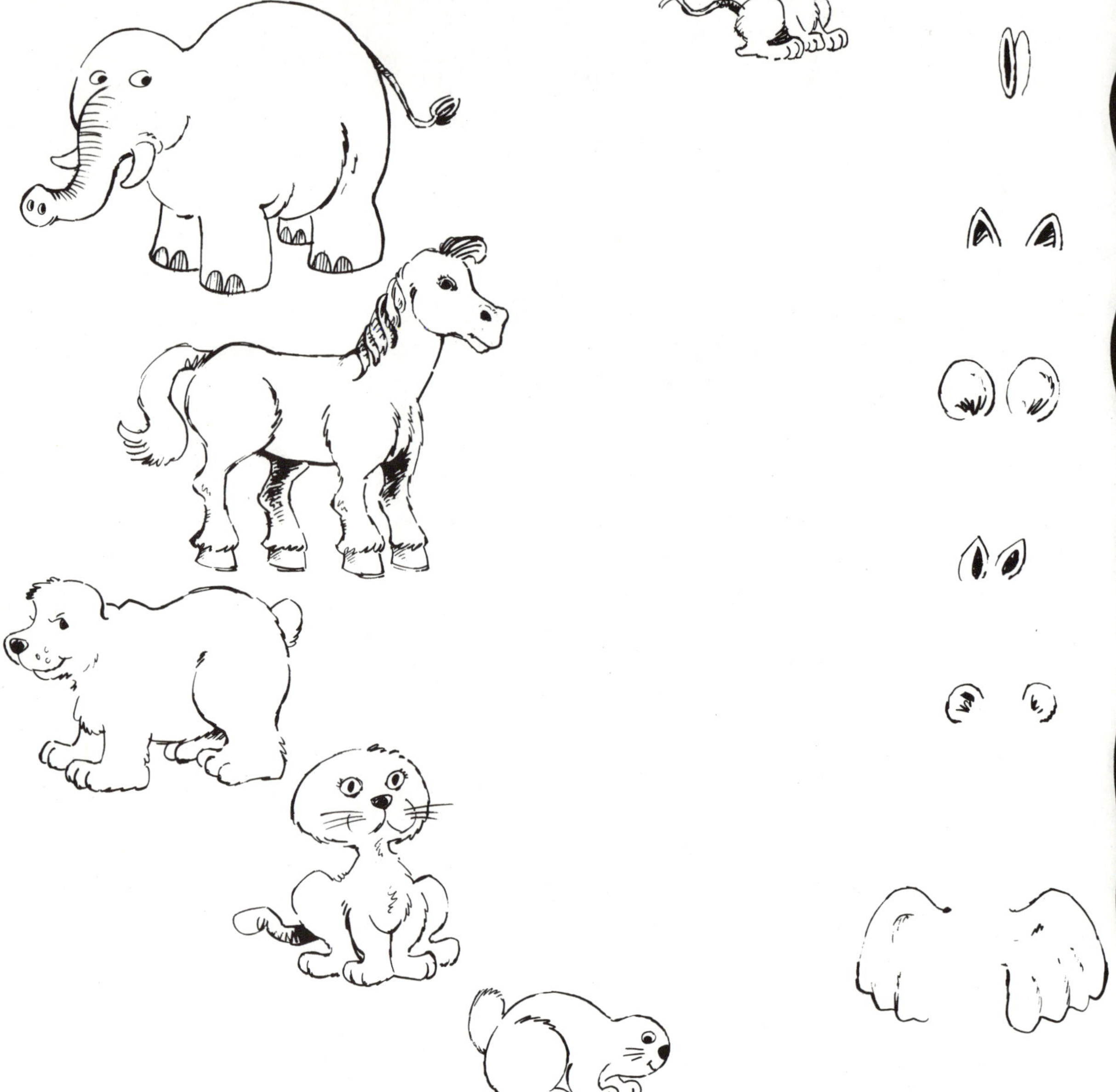

When God created animals, He gave them ears to hear, but they do not look like yours!

The Best Sound of All

The very best thing we hear with our ears is the good news that Jesus loved us enough to die for us and rise again. Through faith we believe in Jesus, receive His forgiveness, and look forward to living with Him in heaven. A new family in town wants to go to church, but they don't know the way. Draw a line through the maze and help the family get to church by listening to the ringing church bell.

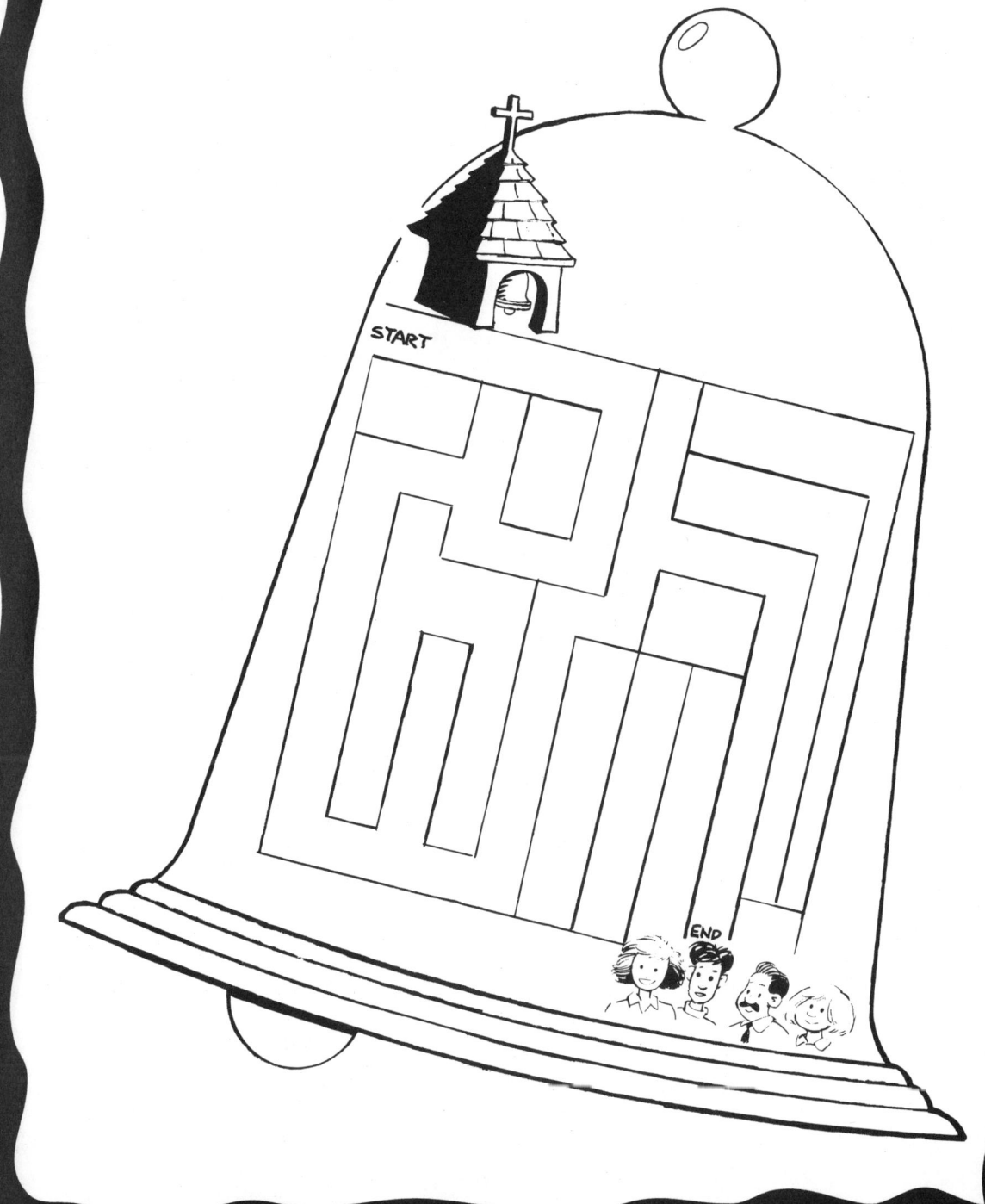

31

Musical Mobile

Materials

Wire coat hanger
Heavy yarn or kite string
4 small tin cans with labels removed
Construction paper
Glue
Markers

Directions

1. Cover cans with construction paper. Decorate with marking pens to make a musical design.

2. Have a grown-up help you clip 18" of wire from a coat hanger.

3. Form wire into a circle and twist ends together.

4. Tie three lengths of 10" yarn or string to wire circle at points an equal distance apart. Gather the top ends of the yarn and tie together to form a hanger.

5. Punch a hole in the bottom of each can.

6. Knot four 8–10" lengths of yarn at one end and thread each length through hole in can.

7. Tie unknotted ends to wire circle. Hang your mobile in a location where it will catch moving air and make music for you.

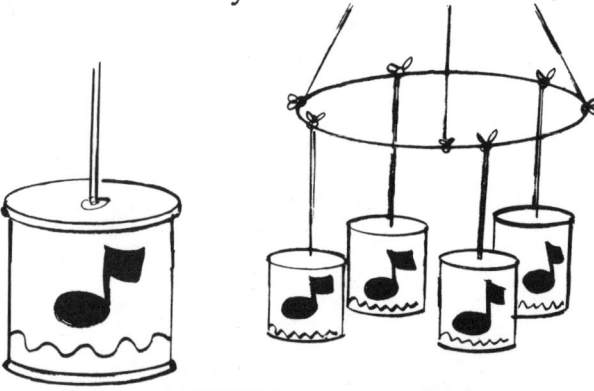